Praise F

Hopeful Heart, Peaceful Mi

"A concise and practical book that helps couples lighten the emotional burden that accompanies infertility. I recommend it to anyone who is struggling to cope with the complex experience of infertility."

—Linda Applegarth, EdD, Director of Psychological Services
Perelman/Cohen Center for Reproductive Medicine
Weill-Cornell University Medical College
New York, NY

"Infertility, like many diseases, impacts you in countless ways—physically, emotionally, and spiritually. *Hopeful Heart, Peaceful Mind: Managing Infertility* addresses these issues in a compassionate manner, and offers couples tools and guidance to help them follow their paths during a journey they most likely never expected to take."

—Jennifer A. Redmond, Editor in Chief
FertilityAuthority.com

"Carol Jones has written an insightful and helpful roadmap to managing emotions and relationships through a fertility journey. She blends her personal experience and professional expertise in a way that is easy to grasp and emulate. She touches on many aspects of emotional care in infertility that are often ignored by patients and their physicians, and provides reasonable remedies for the stress couples face in their quest to build a family. This book is a must-read for patients and for physicians trying to connect holistically with them."

—Dan Shapiro, MD, Director of Egg Donation Services
Reproductive Biology Associates
Atlanta, GA

"While Carol Jones' own journey with infertility is the heart and soul that nurtured this book, it is her professional expertise and long experience counseling couples facing the challenges of infertility that make it such a valuable resource for others."

—Carrell Dammann, PhD, Family Psychologist
Open House, Inc.
Atlanta, GA

"Carol Jones has provided an important book that offers insight and the necessary tools to survive and thrive during your fertility treatment. Readers are advised to celebrate the family and support they have while becoming empowered to build the family they desire. Reading Hopeful Heart, Peaceful Mind: Managing Infertility is a great first step on the pathway to achieving your dreams."

—Mark Perloe, MD, Medical Director
Georgia Reproductive Specialists
Atlanta, GA

"Carol Jones has written an inspiring book; her ability to communicate clearly is evident in every line. Her professional counseling experience and background in yoga teaching make her an ideal voice to speak about this intimate topic and to help those with hopeful hearts find peace when managing infertility."

—Kausthub Desikachar, Cofounder, Krishnamacharya Healing and Yoga Foundation
Chennai, India

"We highly recommend this book to anyone seeking fertility treatment. After eight months of treatment, we felt as though our lives had been completely taken over by infertility. Reading Carol Jones' book helped us feel we could be more positively involved in the process and still take time out for our own lives. It also provided useful stress reduction techniques and ways to approach treatment in a more positive light. Reading about others in fertility treatment also helped us process our own feelings about treatment. This book is like a built-in support group."

—Dan and Nancy, infertility patients

"Carol Jones has a wonderfully positive outlook. We were so fortunate to work with her to confront our emotions and make decisions about our infertility. Infertility caused us to think about what we didn't have in life—specifically, a baby. Carol helped us focus on what we did have. Now, through this book, she offers her helpful approach to others."

—Sheryl and Paul, infertility patients

Hopeful Heart Peaceful Mind

Managing Infertility

Carol Fulwiler Jones, MA

fraser davis press

fraser davis
press

Disclaimer:
The case histories in this book are a product of Carol Fulwiler Jones' clinical work. The names and identifying characteristics of clients quoted throughout the book have been changed to protect their privacy.

Every effort has been made to ensure that the information contained in this book is complete and accurate. The ideas, advice, and suggestions are not intended to be a substitute for seeking professional medical advice. The reader should consult with medical, mental health, insurance, or other professionals as needed. The author is not liable or responsible for any loss or damage allegedly arising from any information or suggestion in this book.

Hopeful Heart, Peaceful Mind: Managing Infertility

ISBN # 978-0-578-02595-7

Library of Congress Control Number: 2009933909

Printed in the United States of America
First Printing: September 2009

Editor: Susan Snowden, Snowden Editorial Services,
www.snowdeneditorial.com

Cover design by Lonnie Busch
Cover illustration used under license from Shutterstock.com
Photograph of the author by Mary Jane Starke

This book may also be ordered on my Web site,
www.TheInfertilityCounselor.com

*This book is dedicated to my sons,
Davis and Fraser. I am grateful each day
for the privilege of being their mother.*

Contents

Introduction xiii

1. Understanding and Supporting Your Partner 1

2. The Illusion of Being in Control 19

3. How to Find Medical Help 31

4. Accepting and Managing Your Feelings 45

5. Family, Friends, and Support Groups 59

6. Deciding Who to Tell and When 71

7. Sexual Passion and Pleasure 85

8. Unexpected Gifts for the Spirit 97

9. Practices for Health and Healing 111

10. Music and Imagery to Enhance Fertility 125

Note to the Reader 141

Glossary of Terms 143

Additional Sources of Information:
Helpful Organizations, Suggested Books and CDs 155

References 161

Acknowledgments

I give heartfelt thanks to the many people who helped and supported me in creating this book. I thank the hundreds of clients I have counseled during their journey to become parents. They are strong and courageous men and women who passionately pursue their dreams. They have been open and vulnerable in sharing their personal stories for this book. Their stories provide hope and inspiration to the millions of people who are affected by the disease of infertility.

I thank the doctors, nurses, and staff of Reproductive Biology Associates and Georgia Reproductive Specialists in Atlanta. It is a privilege to work with the finest physicians in the field of reproductive medicine and to counsel their patients. Particular thanks go to Joe Massey, MD, and to Michael Witt, MD, for providing medical expertise and helpful suggestions.

I am grateful for the wisdom of the Mental Health Professional Group members of the American Society of Reproductive Medicine. Their dedication to providing quality mental health services to infertile clients has educated and inspired me. RESOLVE, The National Fertility Association, holds a special place in my heart, and I am grateful for the support I received from RESOLVE during my own infertility.

Special thanks go to my mentor, Carrell Dammann, PhD. She taught me how to counsel couples, and she encouraged me to finalize the publication of this book. I also thank my coworker, David Rouser, PhD, for patiently listening and offering support.

I have great reverence for my yoga teachers, T.K.V. Desikachar, Kausthub Desikachar, Martin Pierce, and Kathy Davis. Their teachings of Krishnamacharya yoga have provided health, healing, and wholeness to their students. Thanks to Kathy for reviewing the yoga information in this book.

For many years, I have meditated with Liana Carey and Ruth Skaggs. We visualized this book and sought guidance for its creation and publication. Ruth has taught me about classical music and its infinite possibilities for healing and transformation. Her wisdom is most evident in the final chapter of this book. My dear friends Sharon and Steve Paskoff, Millie Lochridge, Janette Gilbert, Gretchen Ventura, D.D. Peters, and Patsy VanDerveer contributed their opinions, criticism, and praise, which were supportive and helpful.

Special gratitude goes to my typist, Mary J. Shipe. Her organization, excellent skills, and attention to details have made my job so much easier.

My editor, Susan Snowden (www.snowdeneditorial.com), has been such a pleasure to work with. Her professional advice and keen editorial eye have been invaluable in the production of this book.

I give thanks for my sons, Davis and Fraser. During my infertility, they taught me how to stay hopeful and patiently wait for their birth. They remind me to live consciously one day at a time.

Hopeful Heart Peaceful Mind

Managing Infertility

Introduction

I am confident that one of my purposes in life is to write this book and share with others what I have experienced and learned through infertility. I have been where you are now. I have yearned to have a baby and felt a profound loss over being unable to have a baby when I wanted to. I have felt your sadness and pain. I felt like I didn't fit in with other women and couples who were pregnant and having babies. I felt my body had betrayed me and that God had overlooked my desire to be pregnant. I now know these are common feelings for anyone who is going through infertility.

For most of my professional career as a psychotherapist, I have had the privilege of counseling individuals and couples who are passionately pursuing their dream of becoming pregnant and parenting a child. I sit with my clients as they share their personal intimacies and private struggles. I admire their courage, strength, and determination as they face the challenges of infertility.

In this book, I have included personal stories and experiences of my clients. They are meant to give you new ways of thinking, feeling, and responding during this journey. In the quotes and stories, I intentionally do not include how the person or couple resolved their infertility. I do not want to mislead you or suggest that if you do what someone else does your result will be the same. Each diagnosis is individual, your responses to medications differ, and your treatment plan is designed for you. You will find your own path to resolving infertility, but you can learn from the wisdom and experiences of others.

I started writing this book in 1991 because I knew I had important and helpful things to say to people who were experiencing infertility. I would periodically write a few pages when I was inspired or motivated. Then I would put the pages away in my "book box" and add to it through the years. When I gave talks on various infertility-related topics, I would add my notes to the box. I have led hundreds of support groups for women and couples, and I would write down their themes, quotes, and helpful suggestions to add to my box. I spent many years listening to, documenting, and collecting stories and experiences of my clients to be woven into this book. Then one day I knew it was time to commit to writing and make the box into this book.

When I was nineteen years old, I had laparoscopic surgery to explore my reproductive organs in hopes of learning why I rarely ovulated. I learned I had polycystic ovaries, and several doctors told me I would have difficulty ever getting pregnant. Since I had no interest in becoming pregnant until I was thirty, these doctors' comments were of little concern to me. Once I wanted to become pregnant and have a baby, I assumed I would have physical obstacles to overcome.

My gynecologist referred my husband and me to an infertility specialist after our initial diagnostic test results. I felt certain this specialist would fix our problem and I would be pregnant within a few months. I never imagined my husband and I would go through several years of medical treatments, which included examinations, ultrasounds, blood tests, oral medications, injectible medications, surgeries, inseminations, and various other medically-indicated procedures.

I experienced a range of emotions during those years, and I stayed hopeful and determined that I would get pregnant. At one point, my doctor encouraged us to adopt, rather than continue in medical treatment. I told him I believed I would become pregnant and I needed his help to do this successfully. After three and a half years, I finally became pregnant with my son.

I wanted another child so I resumed medical treatment with my infertility specialist when my son was one year old. In addition, I decided to work with my body in a more involved and holistic way. I was taking yoga classes and meditation classes, having regular massages, and getting chiropractic adjustments as needed. I had many individual sessions with a psychotherapist who did mind-body work through the use of music and imagery. Each day I visualized my body as fertile and healthy. I continued to see my reproductive endocrinologist monthly. I eventually conceived and miscarried in my second trimester of pregnancy. Two years later, I became pregnant with my second son through in vitro fertilization.

Medical technologies and medications have advanced significantly since I was an infertility patient, and there are many choices available for building your family. This is an important journey in your life, and you do not know where it will lead you. Infertility disrupts your life and you feel a profound sense of loss when your hopes and dreams of having a child are not happening as you envisioned. I wish that everyone who wants to be pregnant would be able to do so easily. However, according to the National Survey of Family Growth, Centers for Disease Control and Prevention, in 2002 an estimated 7.3 million American women of reproductive age, or 12 percent, had experienced difficulties getting pregnant or carrying a pregnancy to term. Two million couples in the United States, or 7.4 percent, were infertile.

Although I mostly talk about heterosexual couples in this book, this is by no means intended to exclude single men and women, gay couples, or lesbian couples who are experiencing infertility. I believe everyone who is infertile should have equal access to medical treatment regardless of their sexual orientation, race, or socioeconomic status. My dream is that one day infertility will no longer be a secret disease and people can openly talk about their treatment and family-building choices without fear of judgment, stigma, or negative consequences. Life is a gift to be celebrated. A child is a gift to a parent, no matter how conception occurs or how a parent and child come together.

Keep this book by your bedside and read one chapter at a time if that is what you need. Some of the medical terminology used in this book may be unfamiliar. If so, refer to the Glossary at the back of the book whenever you need clarification. Practice techniques described in the book to help you feel better and to help you access the healing and wisdom within you. Give this book to your family and friends so they can become educated about infertility and learn how to best support and comfort you.

Infertility changed my life. It wrestled with my soul and my heart, and I reevaluated what was important to me. It became a spiritual journey for me as I explored deeper parts of myself and my relationships with my family and friends. Infertility blessed me with many opportunities to grow, change, and live a more balanced and meaningful life. Take a few deep breaths, begin reading, and celebrate the experiences, challenges, and gifts that infertility offers. Stay aware and curious as the mysteries of your life unfold.

Chapter 1
Understanding and Supporting Your Partner

Your relationship with your partner is a lifelong journey that provides an opportunity to grow with another person and share your passions, your joys and sorrows, your bodies, and your intimate thoughts and feelings. During infertility, you and your partner will experience many challenges, and these challenges can bring strength and closeness to your relationship.

When a fertility problem is diagnosed, you first wonder what this means. You may ask many questions: How serious is the problem? Can it be treated? What will the treatment involve? Can we afford treatment? Do we have the emotional resources to cope? How will our relationship be affected? What are the odds that treatment will result in a live birth? How much should we share with our family and friends?

Infertility treatments may result in a pregnancy or they may not provide clear or immediate solutions. For example, if a man has a varicocele, surgery may or may not affect his fertility. If a woman has laparoscopic surgery to laser endometriosis, the procedure may or may not affect her ability to become pregnant. You may decide to forego recommended medical treatment and either hope for a miracle pregnancy or wait for evolving medical technologies to assist you in the future.

Couples need to communicate their thoughts and feelings with each other. Explore the reasons you want to be parents. For some, it may be to have a legacy and a family after you die. It may be because you want children to care for you in your old age. You may believe that children will give your lives more meaning and joy. Most couples do not question why they want to parent when they become pregnant easily. However, you will have this time to reflect and explore what parenting means to you.

Couples sometimes wonder whether their partner wants to stay married if they are unable to have a child together, and you could be experiencing similar thoughts.

John and Linda are a couple in their early thirties. During one of our couples counseling sessions, Linda talked about how inadequate she felt as a woman and as a wife for not being pregnant. She felt she had let John down and said she would understand if he wanted to divorce her and marry someone who could have a child with him. John said:

> *I didn't choose to be with you just to have a child. In fact, I wasn't thinking of having children together when we were dating and having fun. I chose you for the person you are. I want to be with you whether we ultimately become parents or not. That would just be icing on the cake.*

Men and women respond differently to the stresses and demands during infertility. There is no right or wrong response. Trying to understand and accept each other's differences allows for growth and intimacy in your relationship. You need to communicate openly and clearly with each other so you can understand each other's needs and your different coping styles. Women usually want to talk about their new feelings that surface during infertility. They want to be held and comforted when they feel sad and afraid that they may never be a mother. Give your partner permission to feel whatever way he or she feels. There is no truth to what you "should" or "should not" feel. You just feel what you feel until you feel different.

I counseled Tom and Mary, a couple who were both frustrated with each other. Tom said he was at a loss as to what to say to help Mary feel better when she cried and felt sad about not being pregnant. Tom believed he had tried everything and was unable to comfort her. I asked Mary to tell Tom only one thing she wanted him to do for her when she was crying, and she said, "I just want you to hold me while I cry." He was shocked to hear that was all she wanted, and he agreed to try it the next time she cried. Tom came back the following week saying, "That was easy. I didn't know that was all she needed from me."

You probably know where you like to be touched and how you like to be touched when you want to feel soothed and comforted. When I ask people how they like to be touched in a nonsexual way that feels good, I hear, "I like my partner to rub my back, stroke my hair, touch my face, massage my feet, tickle my arm, hug me closely." The list goes on and on. Ask your partner how he or she likes to be touched. You and your partner probably enjoy being touched in different ways. If you were not raised in a family where loving touch was given and received, you may not like to be touched. In fact, it can feel irritating. If you have a history of being physically abused you might not enjoy being touched. If you and your partner can carefully explore touch together, you may learn to accept and enjoy touch within a safe and loving relationship.

Sue is a thirty-five-year-old woman who has had two miscarriages. She is currently experiencing infertility, and she says:

> *My relationship with my husband has changed in several ways. Although the physical aspect of our marriage needs a little help, the emotional side of things has definitely improved. My husband and I throughout the process became strong. We became two people who had the same goals. My husband always felt so bad because I struggled so much emotionally and he has always been able to be happy with whatever happens.*

Couples may argue during infertility, and they may not agree on treatment plans. For example, one partner may be ready to stop medical treatments and adopt, and the other may want to continue medical treatments. One partner may want to try in vitro fertilization and the other partner may say they cannot afford the expense. One partner may want to use donor eggs and the other may want to stop treatment and live child-free. If Plan A for family building is unsuccessful, can you both agree on Plan B? If these situations arise, it is easy to argue, fight, withdraw, ignore the conflict, and/or give in to the other person's desire against your will.

During infertility you cannot pretend there is no problem, because the issue will not go away until you have a baby, adopt a baby, or decide to live child-free. I do not recommend "giving in" to your partner's desires. Instead, find a way to honor both of your opinions, feelings, wants, and needs. Arguments can be avoided when you better understand what your partner desires and why.

When discussing your feelings, problems, and solutions together, be aware of the tone of your voice and your body posture, understanding that nonverbal communication is often more powerful than words. Ask for what you need and ask for support when you need it. Your partner cannot read your mind and may not be feeling what you feel. Tell your partner how you feel and how he or she can best support and care for you.

You and your partner need to decide which family-building options fit with your belief systems, values, and morals. As technological advances in reproductive medicine are made available, you may become open to medical treatments you never imagined you would consider. You and your partner will need to agree on medical options you will pursue, and it may help to discuss answers to these questions:

- Is intrauterine insemination acceptable to us?
- Is in vitro fertilization acceptable to us?
- Is using donor eggs, donor sperm, or donor embryos acceptable to us?
- If we are pregnant with more than one fetus, is this okay?
- Are we educated about the risks and challenges of a multiple pregnancy?
- Will we tell our friends and family about our medical treatment? If so, how much information should we share?
- If we have a child, will we tell him or her how conception occurred?

If you and your partner do not agree on the next steps in your family building, try this exercise: Each of you make a list of your top three treatment choices. Write down all the pros and cons you can think of for each choice. Take turns sharing your list with your partner and listen attentively while the other person is talking. You may not agree on your first choice, but you may agree on your second choice. Are you willing to compromise in order to become parents? Spend as much time as you need to make this important decision together.

This is the story of Anderson and Jessica, a married couple in their early thirties, and how they made treatment choices:

We assumed we would be pregnant soon after we started seeing a fertility specialist. All our diagnostic tests were normal and we were confident we would be pregnant within a few months if we did inseminations with Clomid (clomiphene citrate). When this did not work, we did four cycles of inseminations with injections. We were comfortable with doing inseminations, but we always said in vitro (in vitro fertilization or IVF) would be out of the question for us. It was too high-tech and too expensive. We agreed we would stop treatment and adopt if we weren't pregnant within a year of trying inseminations.

Now a year has passed and our doctor is recommending in vitro. We would like to have a biological child and we feel we have come too far to stop now. Since we have had so many injections, ultrasounds, and inseminations, in vitro doesn't seem so high-tech anymore. IVF is still a stretch for us and there is no guarantee it will work. If we don't get pregnant through IVF, we will regroup, plan one cycle at a time, and evaluate options as we go.

Many people have difficulty verbalizing feelings. If this is true for you, try writing your feelings on paper or in an e-mail for your partner to read. Reading someone's feelings decreases the emotional intensity since there is no voice tone, facial expression, or body language accompanying the words. Ask your partner to respond by writing back to you. Writing may be a more thoughtful and concise way of expressing feelings because we tend to give our first impulsive and uncensored response when we are talking face to face.

A man may not share his feelings during stressful times, especially if he believes that his partner will be more burdened by listening to his feelings. A man will verbalize concerns about finances and about his partner's emotional and physical health. He often refrains from expressing his emotions in hopes of being kind and considerate of his partner when she is having emotional ups and downs. Then a woman wonders why this is not as emotionally difficult for her partner as it is for her, and communication begins to break down. A woman feels reassured that her feelings are valid when her partner also expresses concerns or emotions.

Peter and his wife, Michelle, have had two in vitro fertilization cycles canceled and he says:

> *The hardest part of infertility for me was when we first found out we couldn't have children. We never imagined this would happen to us. We are generally naturopathic people who don't like to take any medications, and many infertility drugs are used in treatment. My concern is how her health may be affected and how she will respond to the medications. The money is kind of an issue, too, but I am finding ways to afford treatment.*

You do not want the topic of infertility to become the main focus of your conversation each day. If it does, your relationship will seem boring and stagnant. Schedule time with your partner each week to discuss treatment, emotional and physical responses, finances, and future options. When your scheduled time is up, stop talking about infertility and shift to another topic or activity. This structured time is a meeting with an agenda, and this often helps men communicate more openly. This is also a good time to talk about stresses, needs, and intimacy in the relationship. Be sure you also talk about what is working well between the two of you.

A woman begins to feel as if her body has betrayed her each month when she is not pregnant. She may gain weight while on fertility drugs. She may not want to exercise if her ovaries are enlarged and sore, and she may not have the energy to exercise if she is feeling depressed. She is probably not feeling sexy and may not take time to attend to her physical appearance. She is waiting to be pregnant and to buy maternity clothes so she may not be shopping for fashionable clothes. Her focus is on becoming pregnant. As a partner, you can give her support and do things to help her feel better such as giving a gift certificate for a massage, a manicure, or a pedicure. Encourage her to buy a few new clothes regardless of her current weight. Go for walks together after dinner for exercise and do activities together on weekends. Gentle exercise may feel better than vigorous exercise, and exercising together feels supportive and is more fun than exercising alone. Try to be sensitive to her feelings and encourage her to pamper and take time for herself.

Marjorie is a thirty-three-year-old woman who is feeling

depressed and anxious as she prepares for a frozen embryo transfer cycle. We are discussing possible changes she wants to consider making in her life, but she feels unable to make any more changes while she is in treatment for infertility. She says:

> *I am scared to start new work because I am hoping to be pregnant soon. I would have to take time off for maternity leave, and I may decide to stay at home and take care of our baby for a few years. I may lose my insurance benefits if I quit my job, and my insurance pays for a few infertility treatments. A new insurance company would probably not cover infertility as a 'preexisting medical condition.' I'm putting trips and vacations and other fun things on hold. We need to save our money for infertility treatment and don't want to miss a monthly treatment cycle while we are out of town.*

Infertility treatments are not listed in the category of fun, so make efforts to plan fun activities as a couple. If you take trips and vacations together, continue to take them and don't say, "My biological clock is ticking. We cannot take a month off of infertility treatment." A one-month break with no thoughts or plans of treatment can be rejuvenating if you have a positive attitude. It may be exactly what you need to improve the intimacy in your relationship. Sometimes you need to go away together, find your sense of humor, relax, and reconnect.

If expenses limit vacation options, be creative. There are many inexpensive ways to get away and enjoy time together. You can go on day trips, hikes, campouts, or take advantage of weekend specials at hotels. Use the internet travel Web sites to find inexpensive vacations and take time to play together. You can go to the nearest large city and enjoy a new restaurant, attend a sporting event, or spend a day in a museum, theater, garden, or zoo.

A woman usually goes to most of the doctor appointments, but it is important for her partner to actively participate in medical treatment. Even if a man has fertility problems, a woman will have blood work, pelvic examinations, and ultrasounds. She will be the one who has intrauterine inseminations. She will probably take medications by mouth or by injection to produce more eggs and improve the chances of sperm fertilizing an egg.

A woman goes through most of the physical procedures to treat infertility. Since a man cannot become pregnant or deliver a baby, he cannot fully comprehend what a woman feels during these experiences. While you may be equally committed to becoming parents, a woman often reaches her physical and emotional limitations of medical treatments before a man. She may say, "I have had enough. I want to stop." This may mean she wants a break from treatment, or she has reached her limit and is ready to stop.

Robin and her husband, Clay, are attempting a pregnancy with anonymously donated eggs. She says:

I'm the front for all this. I'm the one having daily ultrasounds and taking infertility drugs. I need him to understand and listen to me whine. When he does, I don't feel like I'm going through this by myself at all. It doesn't matter which one of us has infertility problems or who goes through surgeries and treatments because we are in this together. It's 'our' infertility.

Men want to know how to become more involved in medical treatment and how to share the experiences as a couple. To begin with, go to appointments with your partner and stay with her in the examination room. You can hold her hand during an insemination and during an ultrasound. Your input during consultations with your doctor is very important, and you may hear information differently from how your partner hears it.

If your partner needs to take pills to improve her ovulation, you can hand her the pills and some water each morning. You can read the basal thermometer and chart the temperature for her each morning. You can prepare the syringes for injections and give her the injections. You can massage the sensitive injection sites for her after shots.

Reading books or pamphlets, gathering information about medical treatments, and sharing what you have learned shows your involvement. You can tell her often that infertility does not make her less feminine. Men often say they feel helpless and left out of treatment. Getting involved and becoming an active participant gives men more of a sense of inclusion.

Millie has been an infertility patient for three years. She talks about her husband's involvement:

> *He protects me. When I wake up on Mother's Day balling my eyes out, he calls my mother and says we're not coming over. He plans something fun for us to do so we don't feel the pain of not being parents on Mother's Day. He takes care of all the medicine during in vitro and administers the shots. I don't have to deal with all the stress, and that is a huge relief. We learn how to make sure the other is okay.*

It is equally important for a woman to be sensitive to her partner and be involved in his infertility treatments. Figures show that infertility affects men and women almost equally. A woman should go to urology appointments with her partner and participate in consultations. If he has trouble ejaculating for a sperm specimen, she can assist him with arousal or with direct stimulation at home or in a private room at the doctor's office. She can give him reassurance and encouragement during his treatment. She can tell him often that infertility does not make him less masculine.

I ask couples if their relationship has been affected during infertility treatment. Of course, the answers are unique to each couple. Some couples mention financial hardships and sacrifices. Some couples mention emotional struggles. When couples view themselves as intimate and connected before infertility, they often say infertility has brought them closer together. They are sharing a challenging time in their relationship and they are growing stronger together as a result. They want to support and comfort each other.

On the other hand, couples who are distant and not communicating honestly and openly before infertility can expect these difficulties to continue or escalate during infertility. While these are very broad generalizations, intimate couples are more likely to deepen their intimacy during hardships, but distant couples are at risk for further breakdown in communication.

If you and your partner are struggling in your relationship, I recommend you attend to your relationship and assess your strengths and resources before you shift your focus to the pursuit of pregnancy and parenting. There are excellent books to read together about relationships and communication and there are couples therapists to guide and assist you. How well you manage infertility as a couple is usually a continuation of how well you were managing your intimacy as a couple before infertility.

You will both need to take time off from work and arrange your schedule to be at the doctor's office for various appointments. This can be stressful, especially if no one at work knows why you are spending so much time away from the office. You may be constructing stories about where you go when you leave work, and you hope your appointments at the doctor's office will not take long. If you receive disappointing information from your doctor, it is difficult to return to work without feeling upset and worried. Because you are expected to perform at your job, you may try to mask your emotions in your workplace and focusing on work can be difficult.

Listening to coworkers discussing their pregnancies, baby showers, and deliveries may cause feelings of sadness rather than shared joy. Find out if it is possible for you to work from home so you can decrease some of these stresses of being in the office. If it becomes too difficult to balance work, emotions, and infertility treatments, explore the option of working fewer hours. For a small number of women, the stress becomes unmanageable and they request a leave of absence from work or quit their job.

Quitting your job may mean losing insurance benefits, and work meets many of your social, personal, and financial needs. Give careful consideration to how you would focus your time and energy if you quit work. You are putting yourself at risk for allowing infertility to become the center of your life, and staying at home may not give you the meaning and substance for living a happy and full life. On the other hand, some women who have quit work are able to decrease their stress, and have ample time for doctor appointments, exercise, and fun activities. They feel more balanced and healthy.

From childhood, a woman sees other women with pregnant bellies and becomes curious about pregnancy and growing a baby in her body. Men don't share this wonder in the same way. During infertility women are usually more upset than men when seeing pregnant women, which is difficult for men to understand. Men are often irritated with their partner if she doesn't want to be around pregnant relatives or friends or doesn't want to attend baby showers.

Everyone wants to "fit in" with friends, and women may feel left out of the elite group of pregnant women and mothers. When women get together socially, they ask each other personal questions like, "When are you planning to have children? How many children do you have? Are you still seeing your infertility doctor?" These questions remind infertile women of their own pain and loss and feelings about failure to conceive.

If women talk to their friends about their infertility, friends often give unsolicited and unwanted advice about how to feel better or how to get pregnant. When men get together they rarely ask personal questions about a man's sperm count or his infertility treatment. Men will talk about work, sports, and subjects not related to pregnancy, diapers, and breastfeeding. It is helpful for men to understand that these personal questions can be upsetting and emotionally draining for women. Couples can support each other in these difficult situations and try to be sensitive if their partner does not feel like socializing with friends or family.

Richard is a thirty-two-year-old married man who has been in medical treatment for two years. He says:

This has been a mountain for us to climb, and we have taken one step at a time. Infertility has made our marriage stronger. It's made us even closer. Our marriage is stronger than any of our friends', and it is because of how we have handled the hardships of infertility together.

Your relationship does not have to suffer during infertility, and how you cope will be up to you. You are each other's greatest support as you try to build a family together. You are sharing a goal, and the journey, the effort, and the emotional and physical experiences should be shared.

Your relationship requires attention in order for you to stay intimate and connected. Pause when you are leaving home in the morning and look at your partner. Notice their eyes and say something kind and loving to them. Pause again to connect with your partner when you return home in the late afternoon. A hug and a kiss on the lips is more meaningful than a quick kiss on the cheek. Saying, "Tell me something interesting you did today" is more meaningful than "How are you?" Take time to nurture your relationship, care for each other, and have fun together.

Chapter 2

The Illusion of Being in Control

A primary complaint of individuals and couples who are diagnosed with infertility is feeling "out of control." The desire to have a sense of control is extremely important to most people in the early stages of trying to become pregnant. You feel you have no control over whether you get pregnant, and this leaves you feeling helpless and powerless. You also feel you have no control over your body. You want to be pregnant now and your body isn't cooperating. You probably have been able to achieve most things you have wanted in your life, such as completing your education or finding the right job. By setting realistic goals, you can usually work hard to achieve them. It seems unfair that success in pregnancy and parenting has nothing to do with hard work.

The idea of needing medical assistance to become pregnant probably never occurred to you. You knew infertility could happen in other people's lives, but you never imagined it would happen in yours. Conception wasn't supposed to begin with intrauterine insemination on a doctor's examination table or in a petri dish in an in vitro fertilization lab. It is an uncomfortable, unfamiliar thought that conception will not occur during passionate lovemaking in your bedroom. There are plenty of women who do not even want to be mothers and they get pregnant easily or accidentally. This seems more unfair.

Barbara and her partner, Sam, have recently been diagnosed with unexplained infertility. Barbara says:

> *We learned not to take having kids and getting pregnant for granted. We can't control any of it. We've done everything we wanted in life with hard work and determination, but this is unfamiliar territory.*

Infertility might be your first experience with the unsettling concept that you cannot control what life brings you. Life is a mystery and you never know what direction your journey will take. You have no control over when life begins or ends. You may wonder what you do have control over. Did you just imagine that control exists in the first place? Is it all illusion?

You can't make a pregnancy happen nor can you control the timing of many significant events that occur in life. No one is exempt from loss, grief, disappointments, and challenges in life. How you define the meaning of these events is profound and necessary for learning the lessons you are here to learn. They are uniquely your lessons and are about your personal growth and your search for a more meaningful sense of self.

You may be pressuring yourself to be pregnant soon or wishing you were pregnant now. You may not have scheduled this event in your calendar but you have thought about the best time of year to be pregnant or celebrate a birth. Try not to set a time frame for when you will be pregnant. Practice letting go of plans to become pregnant by your next birthday or by the end of the year. Deadlines only put pressure on you, and you have no control over the timing of pregnancy.

For today and every day try not to think of a pregnancy timetable or schedule. Begin to tell yourself that you will be pregnant when it is time to be pregnant, then trust the part of you that believes you will be a parent. Remind yourself each day that pregnancy will happen when it is supposed to. Practicing this reminder daily will lessen your desire to control events and will lead you to greater confidence about becoming pregnant.

You live in a fast-paced, highly scheduled world where tasks are supposed to be completed quickly; phone calls, faxes, and e-mails are expected to be responded to immediately. Waiting for anything you want may be difficult, and you may have developed a low frustration tolerance for waiting. It's up to you to decide the attitude you will have while you wait to become a parent.

Your attitude can change frequently throughout the day. You can respond patiently while striving to achieve your goals in life or you can respond anxiously. When you are anxious, your heart beats rapidly, your blood pressure rises, your palms sweat, your thoughts race, and you may experience a flood of worry and fear. The opposite effects happen when you are calm. What would your infertility experiences be like if you could remain patient and calm? Several tools for relaxation will be discussed later in the book.

You may want to blame someone or something for your difficulty in conceiving. Let go of the blame. It is a waste of your energy. Release blaming yourself for past behaviors, blaming your spouse, and blaming your doctor. There is no blame. You didn't choose to be infertile, but you have complete control over how you choose to respond to infertility. How you manage this ordeal is entirely up to you. You are choosing your attitudes and responses each moment of the day. Be clear about the many choices you do have. You choose how and with whom you want to spend your time. You choose which physician you want to treat you for this disease, and you choose which medical treatments to undergo. Your careful and thoughtful choices will, in turn, influence your responses.

This couple has been in medical treatment for infertility for one year. Jane is thirty years old and has endometriosis. Glen is thirty-one years old. Jane talks about the issue of control, as well as other aspects of their infertility journey:

> *You feel life is a cycle when you go through infertility. In the beginning of a new cycle, I feel hopeful about becoming pregnant. The day my period starts I feel sad. I have no control over this. The only thing I have control over is whether I'm willing to have sex at the right time. I'm in control of the way I react to people. I control taking care of my health. I give the control to God so I don't have to*

focus on this all day.

I become annoyed at God when I get my period. I wonder why some people are allowed to conceive when they abuse their child. We would be really good parents. It's unfair that some people have an easy time getting pregnant and we're struggling. There's no justice. I punish God by not meditating and not spending time with him for a few days. Then it becomes a punishment for me. I tell God about it and then I feel more peaceful. I take care of myself by doing what I enjoy. I eat Mexican food, drink Cokes, and read People *magazine.*

It is difficult to think of your body as "fertile" when you are seeking help for "infertility." What comes to mind when you think of yourself as fertile? What is a fertile life? This is a good time to explore your beliefs about your life and how you can live a more fertile and full existence.

You can choose your attitude about your medical treatment for infertility. Parts of your medical treatment may be uncomfortable or painful, and this is unavoidable. Having blood drawn, pelvic exams, testicular exams, ultrasounds, injections, taking basal temperatures, timing intercourse, and undergoing other diagnostic procedures are generally not events you will look forward to. These procedures will be more tolerable if you tell yourself they are important and useful in determining what medical treatment will best assist you in becoming pregnant.

Think of diagnostic procedures as your ally to assist you,

rather than your enemy to be fought. Imagine your body being strong, healthy, and fertile. Changing your thinking about your body and your medical treatment offers new choices about how to respond.

Begin to pay close attention to your body and listen to what it needs as you go through various diagnostic tests. Learn to trust your body's wisdom and remember you are the expert who lives in your body and knows how your body feels. When you tell your doctor how your body feels, he/she can use this information as a valuable resource for treatment planning. Your body has many rhythms and cycles just as life has an ebb and a flow. Your heart and pulse rates have a rhythm, you have hormonal and menstrual cycles, and you have a breath pattern of inhaling and exhaling.

Your body's rhythms and cycles are necessary for you to stay alive. When you practice paying close attention to your body's rhythms and cycles, you will know what you need to do to feel healthy and balanced. For example, when your heart races, you can slow your breathing and pause from any thoughts or behaviors that cause anxious feelings. You may also be able to detect when you are close to ovulating by noticing if your lower abdomen feels sore near an ovary, your breasts feel tender, or you have larger amounts of clear vaginal mucous. If you are having these symptoms and it has been approximately fourteen days since your last menstrual period began, it is a good time to have intercourse. Note that it is more difficult to detect your ovulation when you are taking oral or injectible medications for ovulation.

Women often report that once they tune into the physical sensations of their bodies, they develop a new and heightened awareness of their physical self. This physical awareness remains long after infertility and fosters a deeper connection to the whole self. Take a few moments now to scan your body and notice how it feels. Do your muscles feel tight or relaxed in particular areas? Do you feel aches or pains? Which part of your body feels most balanced? What feels different when you tighten all your muscles as you slowly exhale?

Margaret recently had laparoscopic surgery to remove a uterine fibroid. She is now trying to become pregnant by taking injectible medications and having intrauterine inseminations. She has been paying careful attention to her body and writes:

> *Since I started listening to my body I can't stop. My body won't let me, and it makes sure I pay careful attention. I'm trying to hear what I am hungry for and eat those foods. I pay close attention to which foods my body craves. I rest when my body feels tired, and I have a regular sleep schedule now. I feel better when I'm listening to my body. I want to try massage and acupuncture. I have already changed the way I breathe and it is more even and steady. I was initially afraid of the future, but now I trust more, worry less, and am more hopeful.*

Use your body awareness to notice whether you experience sexual arousal throughout the day. Tighten your pelvic muscles as you slowly exhale. As you slowly inhale, think of breathing health and fertility into your reproductive organs. Repeat this cycle for many breaths. I often hear clients say they are not interested in sex. Sexual feelings can be enhanced if you focus on your pelvic area, and remember a time when you felt highly aroused. Stay focused on this memory as you allow your body to also remember the arousal.

Your thoughts, feelings, and body all send messages to each other and are interconnected. You may also become aroused by looking into your partner's eyes and touching them in a way that pleases them. You may remember emotions you felt during passionate lovemaking. Your body responds to memories and can recreate sensations you experienced in the past.

You feel your best when you are healthy and living a balanced life. You make decisions throughout the day about your health and your lifestyle. You decide what to eat, whether to exercise, how much sleep to get, and whether you have fun and pleasure in your life. If you do not like the lifestyle choices you make, then I strongly recommend you change them starting today.

You may be your worst enemy when you make up excuses and reasons your life is not the way you want it to be. I assume you want to feel mentally, physically, and emotionally healthy. I also assume a baby wants you to have the healthiest body possible in order to grow and thrive. Take care of your body for yourself, and, hopefully, you will be at optimum health whenever your pregnancy occurs.

A common topic among women in my support group is how they will live differently once they are pregnant. Abby says:

> *Once I become pregnant, I will change the stressful ways I live. I will work less, eat healthy, put my feet up, and relax when I get home from work. I will start exercising regularly and take good care of myself.*

This is not only healthy for growing a baby, but it is also a healthy way of life for you. Why not start living the way you want to live now? You owe it to yourself.

I am reminded of a story written by Ruth, a thirty-two-year-old woman who had been in medical treatment for infertility for over two years. She had polycystic ovaries and had extreme difficulty ovulating. Her husband, Alex, had a low sperm count and had two surgeries to repair varicoceles. They were having intrauterine inseminations whenever she could detect ovulation. Ruth wrote this story about how she decided to take control by changing her lifestyle and taking better care of herself during infertility:

> *When I was in my early thirties, I had a successful career and worked long hours. I was also a full-time graduate student. I had been married for seven years and had an*

active social life with friends. I wanted to be a mother and had been in treatment with one of the top reproductive endocrinologists in the country. I was spending a lot of money each month on infertility treatments. I was highly stressed and always felt busy and rushed between the demands of work, school, and personal life.

I am now aware that this was busyness I created. I was talking to one of my close friends at school one day and said I had to hurry to my doctor's office to be inseminated, but I would be back in a few hours to work on our school project together. He calmly asked me, 'Why do you live the way you live? You are always so hurried and stressed. I wouldn't want your life. Do you really enjoy the way you live?' My first thought was, 'No, I don't enjoy my life and I don't enjoy living in this body.'

My response stunned me as I realized that if I didn't like living in my body, it was crazy to assume that a baby would like living in my body. I decided that day to change some of my lifestyle choices I was making so that a baby might be interested in joining me in my body. Within the next few months, I withdrew from school, worked fewer hours, started practicing meditation, and enrolled in weekly yoga classes. I started seeing a chiropractor and getting massages regularly. I began paying attention to me and the choices I was making. Over time, I began to experience my body feeling healthier and more balanced. My body then felt more connected to my fertility and seemed like a place a baby might want to inhabit.

Infertility may be your first life experience of feeling out of control. There will be others as your life unfolds. Your response to infertility is a significant piece in the character development of you as a person. This may be the foundation for how you will not just survive, but thrive, during other losses in your life. Carefully explore the choices you have, take exquisite care of yourself, and let go of the mysteries of life that are beyond your control.

Chapter 3

How to Find Medical Help

One of the most important choices you will make while trying to become pregnant is finding a good doctor. A recurring theme in my practice is hearing couples say, "I wish we had not wasted so much time in treatment with a doctor who did not specialize in infertility." Your friends, family, coworkers, or neighbors may recommend a doctor whom they have seen or heard about, but do your own research to locate the infertility specialists in your area.

When searching for a doctor, find out if the doctor is an infertility specialist or reproductive endocrinologist. The expertise of reproductive endocrinologists and embryologists varies from clinic to clinic. Some gynecologists do only basic and infrequent infertility treatment but list infertility as a specialty in their practice. Other gynecologists take infertility courses, are serious about treatment, do thorough initial evaluations, and prescribe oral medications. Some gynecologists have been doing specialty infertility work for years and received special training even before the formal board of infertility as a subspecialty existed.

True infertility specialists complete the standard four-year residency in obstetrics and gynecology and continue with two or three years of a fellowship in endocrine training, which includes research. Some of the graduates of these programs never pass the very rigorous academic board exams but are fine clinicians in the field. Other doctors are board certified reproductive endocrinologists and are top of the line as far as credentials go. There are fully trained and qualified reproductive endocrinologists in most medium to large size cities in the United States, and they work in centers that offer IVF (in vitro fertilization) services.

A man may benefit from seeing a urologist or andrologist who specializes in male infertility, and most of these doctors have undergone fellowship training. A specialist in male infertility can appropriately address men's issues or questions, can be a helpful advocate, and can evaluate and treat male infertility problems.

Bill and Connie are a married couple in their early forties. They came to see me for a counseling session and were feeling frustrated and angry. They were referred to me by the reproductive endocrinologist they had seen for the first time the week before. Connie's complaint was common:

> *We went to see my gynecologist after we had been trying to get pregnant for two years and had no success. Our doctor did some hormonal blood testing and because the results were in the normal range, we were told we had plenty of time to get pregnant. We spent a year and a half doing some diagnostic tests and taking seven cycles of Clomid. The doctor never did a semen analysis to check for sperm*

problems.

Friends told us about an infertility specialist they were seeing, so we checked out the doctor and clinic on the internet before we made an appointment. No one ever told us that a woman's fertility starts declining significantly after age thirty-five. I was healthy and having normal periods each month so I never imagined I would have infertility problems. We lost two years seeing the wrong doctor and now my eggs may be too old to get pregnant. If I knew then what I know now, I would have immediately gone to an infertility specialist. Now I know that age matters in being able to get pregnant, stay pregnant, and have a healthy baby.

Several organizations can help you find infertility specialists in your area. RESOLVE, The National Infertility Association, is a nonprofit organization that provides education, support, and advocacy for men and women facing the crisis of infertility. RESOLVE was established in 1974 and has a regional network in your local area. Other organizations are listed in the back of this book.

You can also contact the American Society for Reproductive Medicine (ASRM) to find infertility specialists in your area. Their Web site has a "Find a Doctor" section to help locate ASRM member physicians, reproductive endocrinologists, male reproduction and urology specialists, mental health professionals, and clinics that perform assisted reproductive technologies.

Once you have chosen a doctor who is an expert in the field of reproductive endocrinology, schedule a consultation with the doctor and go to consultation appointments with your partner. The purpose of doctors' consults is to gather information about your medical and fertility histories and to plan diagnostic and treatment procedures. Doctors have unique personalities and their communication skills vary. Although you are choosing a doctor for his or her expertise, it is also important that you and your doctor get along well and are a "good fit." Look for a doctor who:

- Listens to you
- Takes time to answer your questions
- Talks openly and comfortably about the details of your body's reproductive system and your medical treatment plan
- Gives you clear information and explains your disease
- Responds to your concerns
- Allows you to talk about any difficulties you may be experiencing with staff in the office

Paula and Zack changed doctors during their infertility treatment, and Zack talks about their reasons for changing:

We didn't care for our first doctor's style. He talked fast and always seemed like he was in a hurry. He discussed our treatment plan while Paula was still lying on the examination table, and he seemed irritated if we asked lots of questions. We found another clinic and doctor who also had an excellent reputation, and we are lucky to live in a city with several infertility clinics to choose from. Our next doctor took lots of time with us and answered all of our questions. Our consultations were always in his office, which was non-clinical and comfortable. Everyone on his medical team was very caring. We felt they empathized with us and took time to explain things. They were friendly, welcoming, and seemed like top-notch staff.

Some couples refer to their doctor's office as "home away from home" because of the frequency of appointments required. An office that is open seven days a week is not limited in its ability to do ultrasounds, blood work, and intrauterine inseminations. Think of yourself as being part of a treatment team that includes your doctor and the medical staff of nurses, lab technicians, ultrasonographers, and embryologists. You will also have frequent contact with the receptionist and the financial manager in the office. The office staff hopes you will become pregnant and have a positive patient experience.

Infertility is a stressful and emotional time in your lives, so when you see your doctor for a consult, it may be difficult to accurately remember all the information you discuss. This is one reason it is helpful to have your partner with you during consults. If you are like most couples, you feel sad when the woman starts her menstrual period, and the sadness usually lasts for several days. This not only means you are not pregnant this cycle, but you may also need to see your doctor within the next few days to discuss treatment plans for this new monthly cycle. It may be difficult to switch from an emotional space of sadness, disappointment, or frustration to a mental space of decision-making for your current cycle. You may want to prepare for your consultation by writing down questions you want to have answered and bringing them with you to your appointment so you won't leave the office saying, "I forgot to ask about that."

You may also want to:

- Take notes during the appointment if this helps you remember information.
- Keep a log of your treatment, including dates of particular tests or treatments, results, and responses to medication. Review this information with your doctor as needed, especially if your chart is expanding over time.
- Ask for what you need from your treatment team. Each patient has different needs and no one can read your mind.
- Tell your medical team if you have physical discomforts or side effects from medications. You can develop a heightened awareness of your body as you pay attention to physical sensations throughout the day.

- When discussing particular medical treatments, ask your doctor what the success rates are for these treatments. Inform your doctor if you are opposed to trying certain procedures due to religious, personal, or moral beliefs.
- Ask your doctor what the multiple birth rates are for particular treatments. There are many risks associated with multiple births and you should become knowledgeable about potential risks.
- Make sure you have received clear instructions on taking medications. Be aware of possible and common side effects.
- Tell your doctor if you have any allergies and are taking any medications, including vitamins or herbal supplements. Some of these can interfere with infertility medications and should be discontinued.
- If surgery is recommended, find out why. What are the potential risks? Ask about postoperative care, recovery time, and when you will be able to return to work or normal activities.

Peggy and Andrew are a couple from England. They will be receiving donated eggs from Peggy's sister. In discussing their treatment, they say:

When you go down this path you want the best doctor. Infertility is an evolving science, and we want facts and information. Our doctor answers all of our questions and explains our treatment. He talks about the options we may have in trying to become parents. The thing we like most about him is that he is very calming. He is also very positive and says, 'think happy thoughts' when we leave his office. We found everyone in the office to be helpful and friendly. They always remember who we are and that makes treatment easier.

Your doctor is the expert you choose to treat you physically. Ask your doctor to say encouraging and supportive words about your treatment but to refrain from giving you false hope. You want the truth and you want to hear up-to-date statistics for success rates. You also want to believe your treatment will be successful. You create the attitude you will have about your treatment, so why not assume you will be successful in having a baby? You enter into most new life experiences with the intention of being successful. You don't start a new job assuming you will hate the work or be fired. You don't get married assuming the marriage will end in divorce.

Assume your treatment will be successful and try to sustain this attitude. Some couples will become pregnant on their own during a month when they are not receiving medical assistance. While this is possible, do not have an expectation of getting pregnant during an "off cycle."

Couples often say they do not want to get their hopes up for a successful full-term pregnancy because they fear they will be even more disappointed if they do not become pregnant or if they miscarry a pregnancy. You will feel disappointed, sad, and upset if you have a negative pregnancy test or a miscarriage. There's no way around these feelings. However, you will feel better throughout your treatment if you are hopeful that the outcome will be successful.

Many couples who have previously miscarried a pregnancy try to protect themselves emotionally when they are pregnant again. They do not let themselves get excited about this current pregnancy they have worked so hard to achieve, and they don't share their exciting news with family or friends. They deprive themselves of the present joy of pregnancy assuming that this will lessen the pain if a miscarriage occurs. You deserve to celebrate your pregnancy. This pregnancy is from a new egg and sperm and is not the same as your previous pregnancy.

Having one miscarriage does not increase the risk for having another miscarriage, but the likelihood of pregnancy loss increases with age. You will enjoy receiving congratulations from others when you share your great news. If you are pregnant today, celebrate your pregnancy. If you miscarry in the future, you will grieve as long as you need to. The intensity of your grief after miscarriage is separate from the intensity of the hope and joy you can experience during pregnancy.

Your doctor may need to coordinate your care with other specialists or physicians. If a man is seeing a urologist, the reproductive endocrinologist and urologist should be discussing treatment plans and sharing medical information. Sometimes a woman sees her gynecologist for surgery or diagnostic testing because her medical insurance may pay for particular services of the gynecologist but not the reproductive endocrinologist. If so, the reproductive endocrinologist and gynecologist should be discussing your treatment and sharing information. You will need to sign release forms in your doctor's office to give him permission to share information with another professional.

On occasion, a patient lives out of town or will be attempting a pregnancy with a known egg donor, a known sperm donor, or a gestational carrier who lives out of town. If so, the reproductive endocrinologist may need to coordinate some of the medical treatment and care with a physician in another city. This may include blood work, ultrasounds, and medication monitoring.

When choosing a doctor or clinic, you want them to be sensitive to the special needs of infertility patients. Couples hope they will not see friends or coworkers in the waiting room, but other patients are there for infertility also. Most offices request that patients not bring children with them for appointments. It can be upsetting to be around babies and children at this time.

Couples generally view their infertility as a personal and private affair, and it may be uncomfortable to openly discuss your sex life and details of reproduction with your doctor. It may help you to remember that your doctor talks about sex and reproduction with patients all day long, and your doctor can best meet your needs when you can verbalize them. If you have sexual questions or concerns that you are uncomfortable discussing with your doctor, this may be due to your own uncomfortable feelings when openly discussing sex, or it may be that you sense your doctor's uncomfortable feelings when discussing sex.

Our culture is not typically open and comfortable in discussing sex, birth control, reproduction, or infertility. How often did you openly and comfortably talk about sex with your parents? What happened when you talked about sex with your friends? I find that couples often have difficulty talking with each other about their sexual likes and dislikes.

The media today flood us with pictures of sexy men and women, the music videos on television include erotic moves simulating sex, and sex acts are readily available for viewing on television, the internet, in magazines and movies. However, there is little conversation about the emotional component of sex and there is little conversation about sex within the context of a relationship.

The intimacy of sex between two people is overlooked and often portrayed in isolation as a physical act. It makes sense that couples may struggle with intimacy and open communication about sexual desires. If your doctor seems uncomfortable addressing your sexual issues or concerns, ask for a referral to a mental health professional who has training in sex therapy.

To prepare for a semen analysis, the man will need to abstain from ejaculating for at least two days. Typically, the sperm collection takes place in the environment where the man is most comfortable. If a specimen is collected from home or away from the doctor's office, the specimen needs to be in the lab within one hour.

If a man is producing a specimen in the office, he may feel embarrassed and self-conscious when entering a room for the purpose of producing a specimen. He may be unable to relax and focus on becoming aroused in an office where staff is right outside the room. Afterwards, he must give his specimen cup to the nurse or lab technician and pretend that masturbating in a doctor's office is an ordinary and comfortable experience. Ideally, the office will have a private room for men, which usually contains erotic pictures or videos to assist with arousal. You may prefer for your partner to accompany you and assist with stimulation for a specimen, and this is generally encouraged in doctors' offices. The stimulation may be more enjoyable with a partner and another pair of hands can be helpful.

The cost of medical treatment is expensive and many diagnostic procedures and treatments are not covered by medical insurance. Discuss the cost of your treatment with your doctor, because your treatment choices may depend on your financial situation. Talk with the financial person in your doctor's office who can help you determine insurance coverage. Each insurance policy has different infertility benefits, and it is unfortunate that only about one-third of our states have some level of mandated insurance coverage for the disease of infertility.

Contact your insurance company and find out what procedures are covered and what infertility benefits are provided.

Ask if your policy covers infertility medications, ultrasounds, surgery such as laparoscopy and varicocele repair, intrauterine inseminations, and in vitro fertilizations. Ask your insurance agent to send you the terms of coverage in writing. Knowing your insurance benefits will help you with financial planning during your infertility treatment. The RESOLVE Web site also has information about insurance coverage in your state.

It is safest to assume you will be paying out-of-pocket expenses for at least part if not all of your medical treatment. I have known couples who have lived on a tight budget, worked second jobs, or borrowed money in order to pay for medical treatment. Financial hardships can compound the stresses a couple experiences during infertility treatment. Couples should discuss what money they have available to spend on medical treatment. You don't want to spend all your savings, and there is no guarantee that your treatment will be successful. If you decide to pursue adoption later, you want to have the funds available to do so.

It is helpful to periodically redefine the meaning of "success" in treatment. Maybe it means more than whether or not you get pregnant or carry a baby to term. There is success when you feel good about the medical care you have chosen and received. Persistence is usually the key to success, but only you know your ability to continue or stop treatment. Educate yourself and become well-informed so you can understand the rationale for your particular treatment. Then you are empowered to participate actively and cooperatively with your medical team.

It is important to feel that you and your medical team have worked together to make the best possible treatment decisions. You will feel a sense of completion in knowing you have done what you are able to do medically. You want to eventually leave your medical team feeling grateful that you have been treated with respect, dignity, and compassion.

Chapter 4

Accepting and Managing Your Feelings

You will be pushed out of your comfort zone and into unfamiliar feelings during infertility. You may experience a range of emotions and these are probably normal emotions shared by others who are struggling to become parents. Try to be gentle with yourself as you explore new and uncomfortable feelings. Try to be sensitive to your partner, who may also be exploring new and uncomfortable feelings. Feelings show up for a reason, so pay attention to them. All feelings are valuable and sad feelings are as important and useful as happy feelings.

Since your life will be full of both pleasant and unpleasant feelings, this is a good time to practice welcoming the broad range of feelings life offers. Embracing your feelings allows you to live more intensely, more authentically and honestly. If you tell someone you feel happy, this person usually asks why. In order to answer this question, it is common to put your feelings on hold and mentally search for words to explain the cause of your happiness.

No one event causes a feeling. Your feeling is there for many reasons or for no reason at all. For example, a woman often says, "I feel sad because I saw lots of pregnant women while I was shopping at the mall today. Everyone seems to be pregnant or pushing baby strollers except me." Your sadness will stay with you until it is ready to leave, but you encourage it to stay longer if you believe your sadness exists only because of pregnant women in the mall.

April is a woman who experienced infertility after having a child. She says:

> *When I was in my early thirties I had my first pregnancy and my first child. I spent the rest of my thirties trying to have another baby. The longer I was unsuccessful, the more extreme my moods and emotional responses became. My life revolved around being angry, sad, depressed, envious, and tired of it all. Now I am in my forties and things have changed somewhat, but these feelings have definitely not gone away.*
>
> *I don't cry everyday and don't have the intense sadness I felt in the past. I am, however, annoyed every time I hear someone is having a baby. I dislike hearing the stories of how they conceived, how uncomfortable they felt pregnant, how they would decorate the baby's room, and how many siblings this baby would have. I just don't care to listen to these conversations. At age forty-two it still hurts, even though I have stopped trying to get pregnant again. The difference now is that the mood stays for a little while and eventually goes away.*

Your feelings may fluctuate rapidly and frequently during infertility, and the intensity of these feelings often catches you by surprise. You will learn about your range of feelings simply by noticing them. Don't try to stop your low feelings or pretend they don't exist. This is something a man often does during infertility, and his positive intention in keeping his feelings to himself is to ease his partner's emotional burden.

Feelings are an essential part of being human, and you can use them to learn about your inner self. Feel what you feel and notice how feelings come and go throughout the day. Let your feelings pass rather than stay focused and stuck on one particular feeling. For example, if you wake up and take your basal temperature, you may start feeling anxious about whether or when you will ovulate this month. However, you will not stay anxious all day. Notice throughout the day when you feel anxious and when the anxiety is not there. Notice the many feelings you have and become curious about them. You may become more aware of your feelings by asking yourself these questions:

- Where in my body do I feel this feeling?
- What conversations am I having in my head about this feeling?
- If the feeling could talk, what would it say to me?
- Is there something the feeling needs in order to feel different?
- What can this feeling teach me about myself?

Plan on experiencing many emotional ups and downs each month. In the beginning of a new monthly menstrual cycle, most couples feel hopeful. Each month is a new possibility for a pregnancy to occur, so this is a time to be optimistic. This hope usually continues throughout the month, unless the couple hears upsetting news mid-cycle; for example, the woman did not ovulate, the man's sperm was poor quality, or a procedure such as intrauterine insemination or in vitro fertilization was either canceled or had a low probability for success.

If a woman starts her menstrual period, she and her partner feel sad and upset. This low mood may continue for several days and you may cry and not feel like doing social activities. Stay in bed with your partner, rest, rent funny movies to lift your mood, and eat foods you enjoy. Find ways to comfort each other and move through your disappointment together.

Julie is a married woman who has experienced multiple miscarriages over the past two years. She says:

> *I am hopeful each month that I will get pregnant. I take my shots and go with my husband for inseminations. If I'm not pregnant, I am devastated and very tearful. My husband feels just as sad as I do but he doesn't cry—at least not around me. We talk about our disappointment. We used to get so excited and happy if we had a positive pregnancy test. Then we had our first miscarriage and the happiness quickly changed to lots of sadness.*
>
> *There is no way to emotionally prepare for the loss of*

a potential pregnancy each month when you start your period. There is no way to prepare for the emotional crisis of miscarriage. We have learned to be more guarded with our hope and happiness each new cycle now, but being guarded won't lessen our pain and sadness if we miscarry again.

One of the most helpful things you ever said to me was, 'It's going to get better. It always does.' Those words gave me hope, and I say them to myself when I am wondering if my sadness and pain will last forever.

If you are healthy and active you assume your sperm and eggs are also healthy and able to create a pregnancy. When you first hear you may have difficulty getting pregnant, you feel shock and disbelief. You want information about your infertility, diagnosis, and treatment. It is a shock for a woman in her early thirties to learn she is in early menopause and will not be able to conceive using her own eggs. It is a shock for a man to learn he has sperm problems and may not be able to conceive using his own sperm. It is a shock if you are pregnant and learn there is no fetal heartbeat. It is a shock to experience a miscarriage at any time during a pregnancy, and miscarriages are particularly difficult for people who become pregnant through infertility treatment.

On the other hand, the diagnosis of infertility may provide a sense of relief and hope. If you have suspected you have a fertility problem, you may feel relieved to have a confirmed diagnosis. Once you learn about the diagnosis, you become hopeful that the disease can be treated and you can become pregnant. You feel relief and hope once you find a doctor who you feel confident will provide you with expert medical care. You feel a sense of relief and hope when you and your partner make decisions about next steps in family building.

Anger is another common emotion during infertility. You may feel anger towards anyone who doesn't seem to understand how painful and emotionally difficult infertility can be. You may be offended and hurt by insensitive comments from family members and friends. You may direct your anger towards your partner, family members, friends, pregnant women, co-workers, your doctor, yourself, or infertility in general. You are not getting what you want when you want it, and it is easier to be upset with someone else than to sit with your anger. If you give yourself permission to feel your anger, you will notice it often turns into sadness and tears. Tears are healing. Let them flow. Other people generally respond in a more sensitive way to your feelings of sadness than to your feelings of anger.

It is common to worry about whether your treatment will be successful, and worry often leads to feelings of anxiety and fear. The worry begins with conversations in your head about events that you imagine will happen in the future. Since you have no idea what your future holds, you are making up these possible events. When your mind imagines the future, you have the choice to fill this unknown space with positive thoughts or negative thoughts. Negative thoughts trigger worry, deplete your energy, and do not solve your problems.

It is not uncommon to develop sleep disturbances when you worry. You wake up in the night thinking about infertility and the worry begins. Rather than lying in bed and worrying, get up and write down all your worries. Sometimes this can help calm your mental chatter. You can also consciously replace each worry with an opposite and positive thought. For example, write, "I worry about having a miscarriage." Then replace this worry by writing, "I am confident this will be a full-term pregnancy." You truly have no idea how your future will unfold, but you will feel calmer and more hopeful when you create a successful outcome in your head.

If you are having difficulty managing your worry and it is becoming more frequent, you may want to create and structure a "worry time." Schedule ten to sixty minutes each day to do nothing but worry. Say your worries out loud, scream them or write them down, and worry as much as you need to during this time. If worries creep in at other times during the day, put them on hold and save them for your "worry time." Set a timer and stop worrying when your scheduled time is up. Do something else and save your new worries for tomorrow. You will feel more energized when worry is no longer depleting you throughout the day.

Do you ever find yourself asking questions like, "What have I done to cause infertility? What have I done to deserve this? Am I being punished for something I have done?" You may relive negative behaviors, thoughts, and feelings from your past and wonder if they are in some way connected to your infertility. You may feel there is something wrong with your body and wonder if you have caused this disease. You may feel guilty because you spent many years trying to get an education or build a successful career rather than build a family. Be kind and gentle with yourself and find ways to let go of guilt from the past. It may help to talk to a friend, a mental health professional, or a religious or spiritual leader who can help you leave the past behind. It may also help to create a ritual for forgiving yourself and letting go of the past.

Rick and his wife, Morgan, came to see me for counseling during their infertility. Rick says:

> *I wonder if infertility is my punishment for having an unplanned pregnancy with my girlfriend when we were in our early twenties. We always used condoms but she still got pregnant. We weren't ready to marry and we sure weren't ready to be parents. She didn't want to continue the pregnancy and give the baby up for adoption. Our parents said they would support whatever decision we made, and we chose to terminate the pregnancy. This was a very difficult decision for both of us, but I still feel it was the right choice. I haven't thought about this for years, but I think about it a lot now that I want to have a baby with Morgan. The past is behind me and I know in my head that it's separate from the present. I need help letting go of my guilt and blame.*

Rick agreed to create a ritual to help let go of his guilt and blame. He set aside a day for himself to be quiet, still, and reflect on his girlfriend's pregnancy and termination. He wrote all his memories, thoughts, and feelings on paper. After wrestling with various thoughts and feelings, he started to find a peace within himself. That evening he and Morgan burned the papers he had written to symbolize letting go of this event in his past. They bought a special "fertility candle" to light each night before going to bed. As they light this candle, they ask God to bless them with fertility and a child.

Whenever possible, share your feelings with your partner. No two people feel exactly the same but your partner can listen to better understand how you feel. If there are infertility support groups in your area, consider joining one to connect with others who understand and can validate your feelings. You can ask your doctor about support groups in your area. It takes patience, courage, strength, and determination to continue infertility treatments, and you will need support on this journey.

The following letter was written by a woman named Becky who had attended my women's infertility support group monthly for twenty-two months. When a group member leaves the group, I encourage her to write about her group experience so it can be shared with other groups in the future. Becky writes about her feelings during her infertility, some of the lessons she learned, and gives wise advice to other group members:

I will never forget the first time you read a letter that a former 'groupie' had sent after she had her twins. At that point in my treatment, I could not imagine ever being able to write you my own letter. I pray that one of your new 'groupies' will be able to learn from my experience and not give up hope. When I first started coming to 'group,' I was very depressed and unhopeful. There was something inside of me, something evil, I might add, that was telling me that I would never be pregnant. After many months of 'group' and listening to you talk of meditation and positive thinking, I still did not feel any better. I was actually getting annoyed. I saw no light at the end of my tunnel.

After my husband had his varicocele surgery, we went through the typical round of treatments before going through with IVF. I had told myself that I would never subject my body to all of those drugs. The first lesson is: NEVER SAY NEVER!!!!! *I got pregnant during our first IVF cycle, but had a miscarriage very early. After my D&C, my hCG level would not go away, I was sooooo frustrated. I actually can now thank my body for the frustration. Through the months it took for my hCG level to go away, I finally got what you had been talking about for over a year! I started to have a much more positive outlook on everything. There was finally a light at the end of my tunnel. I knew that whatever happened, whether it was having a baby, adopting a baby or being child-free, I would survive the pain and heartache of the last 4*

½ years. It took me spending a weekend with my 3 best friends to make me realize that we all had situations in life and that I would rather have my life and its situations than theirs.

It is easy to say now, but everything does happen for a reason and does happen when it is supposed to happen. My only wish is that I could still come to group once a month! I miss the bonds that I had with you and the other women in the group. Thank you so much for playing such an important role in my treatment. I will always feel infertile. I sometimes have to remind myself when I see a pregnant woman that I have a baby. It is easy for all of the old feelings to overwhelm me even today.

One other thought I would like to share with your new group of women: Whenever you see the pregnant woman at the grocery store that you instantly feel animosity towards, just try to remember that you have no idea what her situation has been. She could very well have been in your shoes not too long ago. When I first tried to have that attitude is when I started to come out of my depression.

I thank you for being such an activist in the infertility cause. I hope one day I can help at least one person as you have helped so many others and me.

Depression and anxiety are common during infertility as you grieve many losses. The following are symptoms of anxiety: restlessness or feeling on edge, easily fatigued, difficulty concentrating or mind going blank, difficulty making decisions, irritability, muscle tension, and sleep disturbance. The following are symptoms of a depression: appetite changes, sleep disturbance, low energy or fatigue, low self-esteem, poor concentration or difficulty making decisions, and feelings of helplessness.

If your levels of anxiety or depression are increasing, it is important to seek help from a mental health professional who can help you manage your feelings and make healthy choices. There are expert marriage and family therapists, professional counselors, social workers, pastoral counselors, psychologists, and psychiatrists who specialize in infertility counseling. Infertility doctors can usually refer you to an appropriate mental health professional in your area.

Find a counselor who specializes in infertility and keeps up with the technological advances in reproductive medicine, the medications and side effects, and the predictable emotions you may be experiencing during this difficult time. Don't waste your time and money trying to educate a therapist who is not knowledgeable about this disease, treatment, and its emotional challenges.

Depending on the frequency and severity of your symptoms of depression or anxiety, you may benefit from medication. This should be discussed with the doctor who is treating you for fertility problems or with a psychiatrist who knows which medications can be safely prescribed while you are trying to become pregnant.

When your life contains a broad range of emotions, you feel more complete and alive. Infertility stirs your feelings and pulls them from deep within you. These inner feelings can be intense and powerful. Be careful not to judge your feelings as right, wrong, good, or bad. They simply are what they are. Notice what you are feeling and use this opportunity to learn about your emotional self. This is the basis for the personal change and growth that will continue to unfold throughout your life. Your infertility path is just one significant part of your life's journey. Feel what you feel each moment and watch the moment fade into the past.

Chapter 5

Family, Friends, and Support Groups

Couples are continually surprised to learn how little their friends, family members, and coworkers understand about infertility. They ask inappropriate questions, make insensitive comments, and say things that upset you and hurt your feelings. You start not answering their phone calls and think of excuses to avoid seeing them. You start isolating yourselves and staying home more so you don't have to see pregnant women and babies. You feel alone. You think no one understands how you feel. If any of this sounds familiar, be assured that these are comments made by most couples who are experiencing infertility. You are not alone. There are over seven million men and women in our country who are infertile.

Mike and Elaine have been through six intrauterine inseminations and three in vitro fertilization cycles. They initially talked openly about their medical treatment with friends and family. However, over time it became too painful to continue talking about their infertility. They say:

> *We don't want to talk about our infertility anymore with our families and friends. They ask us too many questions and it is painful to tell them we are not pregnant each*

month. They keep giving us advice like:

"Just relax and you'll get pregnant. You are under too much stress."
"Why don't you just adopt?"
"If you adopt, then you will get pregnant."
"My friend was seeing an infertility specialist and wasn't able to get pregnant. They went on a vacation, took a break from treatment, and got pregnant. That's probably what you need to do."
"Don't you think you might get pregnant if you didn't worry about it so much?"

We love our family and friends but we are avoiding being with them. We don't want to listen to their hurtful comments and we don't want to hear their advice and opinions anymore. Now we are becoming unpleasant to be around. We have never been this way with our family and friends, and it feels awful.

There are many ways to respond to friends and loved ones. They want to help you feel better and don't know how to do this in a way that pleases you. If they have never been through infertility, they truly don't know what you are experiencing. Encourage them to learn about infertility by reading this book. More importantly, ask them to listen while you tell them what infertility is like for you. You can help them understand what you go through, what you feel, and what you need from them. Tell them to stop asking you questions about your treatment and whether or not you are pregnant, and assure them you will share information when you are ready. Tell them what you want them to say to you and be patient because they need time to practice new ways of responding.

People who love you do not want you to feel sad. They want your pain to stop, and they may have a hard time sitting with your pain. They want to say the right thing to please you and help you feel better. Although you may think they are being insensitive when they say, "Don't worry. You will get pregnant," their intention in saying this is to give you hope, not to upset you.

These are examples of things family and friends can say to you to be supportive:

- Infertility seems stressful. Is there anything I can do to help lessen your stress?
- I don't understand the medical treatments you go through. Is there a book or some literature I can read to learn more?
- You have lots of doctor appointments each month. Would you like me to go with you to some of your appointments?
- I know you have surgery scheduled. Can I bring you dinner that night or help in some way during your recovery?

- I will respect your privacy. I'm here to listen whenever you're ready to talk.
- I understand holidays are particularly hard for people during infertility. What can I do to help make your holidays easier and more fun?
- I've never been through infertility so I don't know what it's like. I want to support you, and it will help if you can tell me what you need from me.
- I hope you will be successful in building your family. There are many treatments to help you become parents, and adoption is also an option. It's not important to me how you become parents, and I will support the choices you make.
- It's okay with me if you choose not to parent. A couple is a family, too.

Melissa is a married woman who has one child. She went through medical treatments for two years but was unable to get pregnant and have a second child. She says:

> *The relationships I have with my family, friends, and co-workers have most definitely been challenged and changed. Thankfully, I still have these important people in my life. My family situation is the hardest because my husband and I are the oldest in our families, and our siblings are still having babies. I am still not a good baby event attender and don't think I will ever be unless it is my chil-*

dren's children.

It's difficult to be a part of daily conversation where everyone is discussing having another baby, confiding whether they want a boy or a girl, how many they want altogether, and how they will decorate the new nursery room. To this day, no one seems to particularly care about my feelings. I find myself making some kind of snide remark or walking away altogether. My family seems to think I've always got a problem, but what they don't seem to ever understand is that I just wanted another baby like each of them. You would think this would be such a simple concept.

As a couple, decide what you need from family and friends. Once you are clear about what you need from them, tell them and ask if they are willing to help meet your needs. Warn them that your needs and moods change frequently and this can be confusing. Friends and family can learn new and sensitive ways to respond to you, and most people welcome your suggestions. For example, tell them that what you need to hear for comfort when your pregnancy test is negative is different from what you need to hear for comfort on the day of your egg retrieval during an in vitro fertilization cycle.

If your pregnancy test is negative, you may want someone to just listen to you, or you may want to hear, "I'm sorry you aren't pregnant. I know you want to be. I am here to love and support you." If you are having an egg retrieval or IVF you may want to hear, "I'm thinking positive thoughts about your cycle. I know how important this cycle is for you. I'm here for you if you want someone to listen or give you support." It requires patience and practice to learn new ways to communicate during the emotional upsets of infertility.

It is usually painful to hear that someone you know is pregnant or has just delivered a baby. You may feel angry or sad when hearing this news because you want to be announcing that you are pregnant or having a baby. You feel left out of the world of fertile men and women, and now your life seems inundated with pregnant women, babies, and children. You notice them at work, at the mall, at restaurants, at your place of worship—everywhere you go.

You begin to avoid being with people who are having conversations about pregnancy, and you certainly don't want to hear pregnant women complain about their physical discomforts. You would welcome the opportunity to experience morning sickness and would be thankful for a pregnancy. If a friend calls to tell you she is pregnant, you wish she had not told you; yet if you hear from someone else that your friend is pregnant, you wonder why your friend didn't call and tell you this news. You don't know how or if you want to hear that a friend or relative is pregnant, and the pregnant person is also at a loss as to what to say to you. Keep in mind that most people don't know you are having difficulty getting pregnant, so they are not aware that pregnancy is a sensitive topic for you.

There are many ways to respond when you hear that a

friend or family member is pregnant. An example is, "Congratulations. That's exciting news for you. I also want you to know this is difficult for me to hear because of my own struggles with getting pregnant." If face-to-face conversations are too difficult, you can leave phone messages when you know no one will be home to answer the phone. You can also send a note, a text message, or an e-mail to express congratulations.

Don't go to baby showers when you don't feel up to it. You can send a gift or bring a gift before the shower with a note saying, "Sorry I am unable to come to your shower. Have fun." You don't owe anyone an explanation of why you are not able to come, so make plans to do something enjoyable with your partner instead. Shop for shower and baby gifts through catalogues or on the internet to avoid going into baby stores.

If you are with people who are talking about pregnancy or babies, you can leave the room if you feel uncomfortable. If you are at a party and don't feel like being there anymore, you can choose to leave. If someone asks why you are leaving, simply say, "I don't feel well." Your feelings are emotional, as well as physical, and no further explanation is required. If you are at work and the topic of babies or pregnancy starts, go outside for a walk. You will need to find many ways to take care of yourself when you feel sad or upset, and you are the person who knows best what you need.

Carefully choose the friends and family you want to include in your life at this time. Surround yourself with people you trust to care about you, love you, and support you. You are asking those around you to be flexible with your mood fluctuations, be patient, and stay connected to you as you move through the ups and downs of your hopes and disappointments.

If you withdraw from others and isolate yourself, you will probably feel more alone and misunderstood. Connect with others who are experiencing infertility by going to support groups. Internet chat rooms or infertility Web sites can be helpful if you are seeking emotional support, but be aware that the medical information exchanged is not always accurate or applicable to your diagnosis. This is also a perfect time to be alone with your partner, be romantic, enjoy sex, and have fun together.

Hopefully, you will grow and change every day of your life. In this process, new friends will come into your life and some old friends will exit. You will learn new information about yourself and about your friendships during infertility. As a result, you may let go of some relationships that no longer work in your life. Clearing out friendships that drain your energy can bring a sense of freedom and allow space for new, positive friendships to develop.

One of my clients with infertility said, "Some of my friends were so good to me during this time and some will never get it. I do have some friends I parted ways with because they did not know how to handle me and I could not handle them." Today and throughout your life, take care of yourself by choosing to be in relationships with people who are loving, compassionate, and able to meet your needs.

Joining a support group can be helpful for men, women, and couples who want to explore family-building options, as well as those who are experiencing stress during medical treatment, secondary infertility, or pregnancy loss. Groups for people considering using surrogates or egg, sperm, or embryo donors are helpful in exploring specific issues related to third-party reproduction. The group leader should be licensed in your state, specialize in infertility counseling, and be trained in group therapy. Since people often feel isolated, alone, and misunderstood during infertility, there are many benefits of connecting with others and receiving comfort and validation that what you are experiencing and feeling is normal.

I have led hundreds of support groups for couples and women who are experiencing infertility. At the first group meeting, I ask group members what they hope to get out of being in our group. These are some of their answers:

- *To not feel so alone*
- *To meet others going through the same thing*
- *To learn ways to deal with pregnant people*
- *To find relief from frustrations through discussion*
- *To reach a peace of mind and come to terms with my situation*
- *To address my fears*

Groups provide an opportunity to express your thoughts

and feelings openly and in a safe environment. Your group leader and other group members will suggest new ways to cope in difficult situations. You will talk about healthy ways to respond to others, how to take care of yourself, and how to make decisions about next steps and family building. Although you are not required to talk in groups, the more you participate, the more you will benefit. In my ninety-minute group meetings, we spend the first hour discussing various topics. Then the last thirty minutes are spent practicing relaxation techniques, breathing exercises, yoga, or music-evoked imagery. These experiential techniques are designed for personal exploration and stress reduction.

After a group meeting, I occasionally ask group members what they found to be most useful during the group. These are some of their responses:

- *Being able to laugh and cry with others*
- *Learning from other group members*
- *Sharing and validating the feelings I have*
- *Learning about in vitro fertilization from someone who has already done one*
- *Hearing other people's problems and realizing how similar they are to ours*
- *Open discussions and flow of information from everyone*
- *Listening to others at different stages of dealing with infertility*
- *I feel I will go into egg retrieval tomorrow with a more*

positive attitude.

- *I have struggled with feeling bad about myself. This has helped me to understand that I am normal to have the feelings I do. Although it is usually difficult for me to talk to complete strangers, I was able to talk freely without getting upset.*
- *I wasn't sure what to expect. I was pleasantly surprised. The women in the group seemed very sincere.*

As you begin to open up, relax, and feel more positive about your life, infertility seems easier and more manageable. Being part of a group is an opportunity to get to know yourself, shift your feelings, and make changes in your life. Receiving comfort, support, and understanding seems to bring a peacefulness and ability to cope with your situation no matter what the outcome. One day you will no longer pay much attention to whether women around you are pregnant. One day your friends will no longer be getting pregnant and taking care of infants. One day this time in your life will have become part of your past.

Chapter 6

Deciding Who to Tell and When

Most couples view infertility as a private experience. They may feel uncomfortable, embarrassed, or ashamed to discuss their infertility with family or friends. They struggle with whether to keep aspects of infertility evaluation and treatment confidential or to share this information with certain family members and friends who have been sensitive and supportive. This is a common dilemma for many couples, and there are important relationship dynamics to consider.

You know how you communicate with your family, and you know which topics are discussed openly and which topics are avoided. As a couple, talk about family members and how you think they would respond to hearing about your infertility treatment. How do they usually respond when you tell them something personal? Do they listen, ask questions, give opinions, or offer support?

I ask couples if they have discussed their infertility with any family members or friends. I am also prepared for the conflicts that often occur as they answer this question. One person in the relationship may have been discussing infertility with close friends and the partner assumed this was a private, personal issue that would not be shared with anyone. With guidance, the couple is able to communicate, compromise, and agree on which people, if any, they choose to share their infertility with. It is important to find comfort and support as you are trying to have a baby and this can be given by your partner, your medical team, a friend, a family member, or a mental health professional with infertility experience and training.

Frank and Lisa have been trying to become pregnant. Frank recently had varicocele surgery in hopes of improving his sperm count. A few months after surgery, they began intrauterine inseminations. They say:

> *We are very close with our families, but we don't know whether to tell them about our infertility treatments. We know they want grandchildren and we feel like we are letting them down. This is upsetting to us and we don't want them to worry so we haven't told them anything yet. It seems like we are keeping a secret because our families have always talked openly about problems. We know how much our families love us, and we could use their support now. There are pros and cons for sharing our infertility with our families, and we need help in deciding what to do.*

Couples also struggle with how to answer these questions from people they meet:

- Do you have children?

- How many children do you have?
- Do you want children?

When someone asks these questions, they are typically trying to be friendly and make conversation. People you meet don't intend to cause you pain or discomfort when they ask questions about children. However, these questions can be painful, especially when you are not expecting them and are not sure how to answer them. You are not obligated to give an explanation. Simple answers such as, "Yes, "No, "None," "Maybe," or "Probably" are sufficient. If you feel compelled to say more, you can say:

- *We will have a child when our bodies cooperate.*
- *We are trying and hope to be parents soon.*
- *Having children has not been easy for us. We are hoping to be parents one day.*

If you get pregnant and have a baby through insemination or through in vitro fertilization with your own eggs and sperm, you may or may not choose to tell your child how conception occurred. Many couples see this as a non-issue and do not believe this information would have negative psychological or emotional effects on their child. In fact, many couples want to share this information with their child so the child will know how much he/she was wanted. A child may feel even more special after learning about the medical treatment you went through.

Couples prefer to have a child using their own eggs and sperm, but this is not possible for everyone. There are many physical and medical reasons why a woman may not have the option of using her own eggs to conceive, and why a man may not have the option of using his own sperm to conceive. They may want to avoid transmitting a serious genetic disease. In addition, many single men and women want to be parents. Many same-sex couples want to be parents. In order for this to happen, they may need to use donor eggs, donor sperm, donor embryos, or a surrogate uterus.

Using anonymously donated sperm with insemination began in the 1950s, and in 1978 the first child was born from in vitro fertilization. Once IVF technology was available, eggs could also be retrieved from donors, and embryos could be transferred into the uterus of a gestational carrier. Anonymous egg donation began in 1983 and has been widely used since the early 1990s. Anonymous embryo donation is now available from couples who have gone through in vitro fertilization, have completed their family, and want to donate any remaining frozen embryos to an individual or couple.

Kim has an elevated FSH level and has not been able to get pregnant. She and her husband are planning to attempt a pregnancy with anonymously donated eggs. When asked how she feels about using donor eggs, she says:

> *I'm okay with it now. Initially, I was very sad and angry. I*

am only thirty-three, and I felt like I was doing everything right. I felt like God was punishing me. After a while I accepted it. I did acupuncture, yoga, and special diets. All that stuff made me feel better, but it didn't change my FSH level. Then I decided to get proactive, took control, and felt better mentally. I am willing to do whatever I have to do. I want a baby. I want to be a mom. However I get pregnant, I know I'm going to love our baby.

These are quotes from men who are attempting to have a child with anonymously donated eggs:

- *It took a while for me to reconcile myself to the donor egg scenario. Our goal is to have a family. I would rather have a child that at least has my genetic components. In my mind, this is the best option.*
- *I have always thought I would get married and have children. I prefer to have a child using her eggs, but I have accepted that this isn't going to happen. I'm excited about this opportunity to experience pregnancy and delivery together.*
- *I researched all the options and the statistics. Once I understood the process I was comfortable with it.*

These are quotes from women who are attempting pregnancy with anonymously donated eggs:

- *Having a child is most important to me and I can't have a child with my own egg. I want a child to raise, love, and educate.*
- *The baby is going to grow inside me. I have never been hung up on the genetics of having a child. I just want to be a mom and raise a child.*
- *I have always thought I would be a parent but I never met anyone until now that I wanted to spend my life with. I'm bummed about using donor eggs but this way I am taking care of myself during pregnancy. It's my husband's sperm and that's important to him. I'm real close with my nieces and nephews and we want to have a family of our own.*

Mattie is a single woman who is attempting pregnancy with anonymously donated sperm. She says:

> *When I was thirty-seven years old it seemed as though I wasn't going to meet anyone to be in a relationship with. Most guys my age are married, or divorced and already have children. I kept hoping I would meet the right person to have a baby with, but I never did. Time is running out for me to be fertile and it may have already run out. I am financially stable and have great support from my family and friends. Everyone knows I want to get pregnant, and I am looking forward to this. It would be my dream come true. If I'm not successful, then I plan to adopt.*

An anonymous donor may never know whether a pregnancy ever occurred as a result of their donation because it may be clinic policy not to disclose this information to a donor. Although a donor's intent is to help the recipient become pregnant and to receive financial compensation, many donors would like to know whether a pregnancy resulted from the time and effort they committed during the donation cycle. Other donors simply desire to help and give to others and prefer not to know the outcome.

Elizabeth wants to be an anonymous egg donor. She has one daughter and would like to have another child in the future. When asked how she made the decision to be an egg donor, she responded:

> *I love my daughter so much and she is such a blessing. I wasn't trying to get pregnant with my daughter, but she was trying to come into my life. I have a lot of infertility in my family and there has been a lot of sadness about not being able to conceive. I want to help someone get pregnant who is not as fortunate as me.*

If you have a child through donor sperm, donor eggs, or donor embryos, you may struggle with the issue of whether to eventually tell your child how conception occurred. Couples often think they don't need to make this decision before they are pregnant, but this issue should be given careful consideration. This decision can affect your personal life, your marriage, and the life of your unborn child. Can you tell your child how his/her conception occurred and not share this information with family or friends? Absolutely. In fact, the more people that know about this, the more likely it is that your child could hear this information from someone else.

Parents want to be in charge of disclosing this important information to their child. It is important for both you and your partner to agree on whether or not to tell your child how conception occurred. If you do not agree, you may give your child mixed and confusing messages when he/she begins to ask questions. Couples ask, "What is the right thing to do?" and "What is best for the child?" The Ethics Committee of the American Society for Reproductive Medicine states in their *Journal of Fertility and Sterility,* "While ultimately the choice of recipient parents, disclosure to offspring of the use of donor gametes is encouraged." Honesty in families works best. Otherwise, you will guard your secret and live with the worry that your secret may be discovered.

If you are considering using donor sperm, donor eggs, or donor embryos and you want to explore whether to tell your child how conception occurred, these are some things to think about:

- Are you usually an open or closed person when it comes to sharing personal information?
- If you were conceived with donor eggs, donor sperm, or donor embryos, would you want to know? Why or why

not?

- Do you believe your child has a right to know how his/her conception occurred? Why or why not?
- Are you comfortable telling your child about your infertility? Why or why not?

Dray and Betsy are a couple attempting a pregnancy with anonymously donated sperm. When asked whether they would want to tell their child how conception occurred, Dray said, "I would want to tell. A child should know the details of his origin. I think it's inevitable our child will find out one day." Betsy says, "I'm not sure if it matters whether the child knows or not. I would like to be honest and open, but how do you tell and when?"

Most people wonder how and when to tell their child about donor conception. Reproduction is more fully understood when we become mature adults, but if you don't tell your child how conception occurred until her adulthood, she may be angry and upset that you did not tell her about the donor earlier. While teenagers have some grasp of reproduction, they are moody and are exploring their own sexuality and identity. They also like excuses to be mad at their parents, and this could be a good excuse. So, when do you tell your child? Begin your story when your child is young and add to it as your child is developmentally and emotionally able to understand more details about reproduction.

When children are between the ages of three to six, they

often notice pregnant bellies and babies and try to understand the connection between pregnancy and birth. Your child may ask, "Where do babies come from?" or "Where did I come from?" This is an ideal opportunity to say something like, "I'm glad you asked. We really wanted to be your parents, so we found people who could help us get pregnant with you. We found a nice doctor and a nice lady (if egg donor) who helped us. We are so blessed to be your parents." You probably also have pictures of your pregnancy and of your baby to share with your child.

The next logical time to add more information is when your child is between the ages of nine and twelve. Girls are starting menstrual periods and boys are developing preadolescent bodies. Children this age are more curious about reproduction and about their own changing bodies. As they ask questions, it's a good time to fill in information about the "nice lady" who helped you get pregnant. As your child becomes curious and asks more questions, answer the questions openly and honestly. Give your child information that he is able to understand at his present stage of development.

People will notice your pregnant belly but it does not occur to them to question, "Whose egg and sperm created your pregnancy?" This is one reason some couples do not believe it is important to tell their child how conception occurred. There are various reasons you may not want to disclose this information to your child. You may believe your child would be treated differently by family, friends, or your community if others knew about donor conception.

You may not have worked through your own feelings about your infertility; therefore, it would be difficult to share this with your child. You may come from a culture or a religion where donor conception is not accepted. You may not see the point in telling a child who probably will not have access to information about the donor other than what you were told by your doctor, clinic, agency, or sperm bank.

Gather as much information about the donor as you can because it may the only information you will ever have to share with your child. Your child may have some questions about the donor or the donor's family, including offspring, that may never be answered.

If you choose not to disclose to your child how conception occurred, it is not recommended that you share this information with other family members or friends. They could unintentionally tell someone, and this information could be given to your child. If you choose not to disclose to your child that conception occurred with a donor, keep in mind that your child may be quite upset if he finds out through someone else, through DNA testing, or through expert internet skills. You will have shaken his foundation of safety and trust in you, and he would want to know why you did not tell him. He may also wonder if you have withheld other important information about your family.

There is no absolute guarantee of privacy in medical records or with medical personnel. The staff in your ob-gyn office has access to your medical chart and so does your insurance company. Ask your ob-gyn not to write in your chart that conception occurred with a donor. While it is probably important for your ob-gyn to know that conception occurred with a donor, tell your doctor that you will mention this at all of your appointments but you do not want this information written in your chart.

You will also need to weave the donor's family medical history into your own family medical history. You do not want to be in an emergency room with your child one day and wonder whose medical history you should give to assist the doctor in diagnosing and treating your child.

If you are unable to carry a pregnancy full term, you may find a surrogate to carry a pregnancy for you. Sometimes a friend or family member offers to be a surrogate, and surrogates can be found on several internet Web sites. An attorney who specializes in third-party reproduction and adoption may also be a good resource for finding a surrogate. Surrogates are either gestational carriers or traditional surrogates. A gestational carrier becomes pregnant with embryos created through in vitro fertilization using the egg and sperm of two other people. She carries and delivers the baby for the intended parents.

The second type of surrogate is a traditional surrogate who uses her own eggs to conceive through intrauterine insemination or in vitro fertilization. She carries and delivers the baby for the intended parents. Due to the unique relationship that intended parents have with their surrogates, they may continue having contact with each other after the baby is born and sometimes for the rest of their lives. Intended parents usually tell their friends and families about the surrogate who is carrying their child. They usually tell their child about the surrogate, too. Since the surrogate is obviously pregnant, she tells her friends, family, and her own children that this is not her baby, but she is pregnant with another couple's baby and will deliver their baby for them.

This is a quote from a married woman with two children. She is planning to be a gestational surrogate for a couple who has miscarried several pregnancies:

> *I saw a television program about a couple using a surrogate. The couple had several miscarriages and couldn't carry a pregnancy. They suffered so much and went through so many infertility treatments. This was very sad for me to watch. I am healthy and got pregnant easily with my babies, but many people can't do this. I like being pregnant and it's easy for me. I wanted to help somebody have a baby so I started surfing the internet. My husband and I talked about this a lot and he searched the internet with me to learn about the surrogacy process and the risks. We talked about how it will affect us, our family, and the other couple. We think this is a great thing to do for someone who can't have a family. We enjoy our children so much and I would be so proud to have a baby for someone else.*

You may wonder if your child will still think of you as the "parent" if he knows conception occurred with a donor or surrogate. A "parent" is the person who lives with and cares for a child each day of his life, and obviously a child knows who raises and parents him. Children emotionally receive information the way the parents emotionally give information, so if you are comfortable telling your child about her conception or gestation, then she will probably be comfortable hearing this information as well. When you sincerely tell your child she is special and loved and you treat her accordingly, then she will feel special and loved. This love comes from you as a parent, not from a donor or surrogate who assisted in the conception or gestation of your child.

CHAPTER 7

SEXUAL PASSION AND PLEASURE

Couples want to stay connected during infertility, and they do not want to settle for mediocre sex. They want to please each other and rekindle the enjoyable sex they shared before infertility. They want to get back into the rhythm of having sex. Satisfying sex is different for every couple, and you and your partner cocreate ways to keep your interest and passion alive.

Your sex life may be disrupted and challenged during infertility diagnosis and treatment. You have probably grown up assuming you would be a parent one day. You heard about infertility but never imagined it would affect your life. During the preteen years you started to learn about reproductive organs, how pregnancy occurs, how to prevent sexually transmitted diseases and unwanted pregnancy, and what to expect as your body matures.

As you began to explore your body, either by yourself or with a partner, you discovered sexual arousal and pleasure. If you didn't get pregnant after you were having sexual intercourse, you were either using birth control to prevent pregnancy or you thought you were "lucky." Now you want to be pregnant and aren't feeling lucky if you have been having unprotected intercourse for a year and are not pregnant.

The frequency of intercourse and the level of desire for sexual activity varies among couples. It is influenced by many factors such as travel, sleep, stress, and health. Emotions associated with shame, guilt, low self-esteem, or depression may affect your sexual arousal. Certain medications can have side effects of decreased sexual desire and decreased sensation with sexual stimulation. You may have intercourse every day or once a month. If you have low sexual desire, it does not necessarily mean you have difficulty becoming sexually aroused. You can probably remember times you were not interested in having sex, but if your partner approached you seductively and touched you in stimulating ways, you became interested and sexually responsive.

You are capable of shifting your sexual interest or desire. If you want to increase your sexual desire, first become aware of your desire to be close to your partner. What memories, thoughts, feelings, or fantasies come to mind when you do this? Picture in your mind a particular sexual experience with your partner that was pleasurable and satisfying. You may find your sexual desire increasing as you do this and you may want to share the memory with your partner. Once you are able to feel desire for your partner, the next step is to respond to this desire by touching and allowing arousal to build.

You will not hear couples say their sex life improves during infertility treatment. Instead, they report that their sexual activity ranges from "about the same" to nonexistent. The mental, emotional, and physical experiences of infertility can have a negative impact on your sexual desire. You may find your sexual desire decreasing as the focus of sex shifts from pleasure to becoming pregnant.

Couples often lose interest in having sexual intercourse except during the middle of the woman's menstrual cycle each month when she is most likely to become pregnant. Knowing you have a one- or two-day window of time each month when a sperm can fertilize an egg is stressful and puts pressure on the couple to have intercourse whether they feel like it or not.

If you are trying to get pregnant on your own without medical assistance, you should have intercourse more frequently between seven and twenty-one days after the woman's menstrual period begins. You can buy ovulation predictor kits at the pharmacy to help determine when the woman will be ovulating, or releasing an egg from her ovary. This is indicated by a hormone change that shows up in urine.

If you are planning intercourse around ovulation or seeing a specialist to diagnose why you aren't getting pregnant, you may begin to think of sexual intercourse as something you are required to do rather than something you want to do. In addition, this can affect how you perceive your masculinity or femininity. You may not feel sexy or desirable and you may assume your partner doesn't find you desirable. This is a good time to talk about these feelings with your partner, rather than assume your partner thinks and feels the same as you.

It is not uncommon for a man to experience sexual performance anxiety or erectile dysfunction when he is required to have an erection and ejaculate. This can also occur when a male needs to produce a sperm specimen for intrauterine insemination or in vitro fertilization on the day the woman is ovulating. Since the woman has probably been on oral medications or injections to produce more eggs in preparation for insemination or in vitro fertilization, this sperm specimen is extraordinarily important.

If a man has difficulty becoming erect or maintaining an erection, it helps to remember that this is a common physical response to the psychological and sexual pressures of infertility. He may want to discuss erectile dysfunction with his infertility doctor, and if the doctor decides that taking medication is safe and medically indicated, a prescription for Viagra, Levitra, or Cialis could help. These medications increase blood flow to the penis when a man is sexually stimulated and can help him get and keep an erection for satisfactory sexual intercourse or for producing a sperm specimen.

Sometimes if a man is having erectile difficulties, he may become more aroused if he focuses on sexually pleasing his partner. Excitement for a man is receiving pleasure, as well as knowing he is pleasing his partner, and a woman can be pleased in many ways besides having intercourse.

William and Susie are a couple in their mid-thirties who are attempting a pregnancy with intrauterine insemination. They say:

We have a strong marriage but it has taken a beating

during infertility. Sex has become very scheduled and not spontaneous at all. We started thinking of sex as what we do when we are trying to become pregnant. We used to enjoy having sex. Now we are rarely in the mood, so we can take it or leave it. Our doctor has told us not to have sex for two days before an insemination so sperm can build up. Since we are not very interested in having sex anyway, these two days of having no sex have gradually turned into weeks of no sex. We feel closer when our bodies touch and connect physically. We need to give sex special attention during our infertility treatments.

Since infertility treatment is for a disease of the reproductive system, medical treatment can inhibit the pleasurable feelings associated with sex. A woman may experience hormonal fluctuations while taking fertility medications, and hormones may affect her moods. Sometimes when a woman is taking hormones, she feels balanced and is more interested in sex. For some women, the opposite can occur. Hormones may also contribute to weight gain, which may leave a woman feeling sexually undesirable. Emotional states such as anxiety and depression will also decrease your interest in sex.

A couple's normal sexual activity is interrupted during diagnostic testing, treatment, or when a woman feels physical discomfort. Sometimes when a woman is taking oral or injectible medications that stimulate the ovaries to produce more eggs, her ovaries become enlarged and intercourse can be painful. If so, it helps to experiment with various positions during intercourse, have gentle intercourse, or find sexual satisfaction without intercourse.

If intercourse is painful due to enlarged ovaries, a more comfortable position during intercourse is for a woman to lie on her back with a pillow under her hips so the pelvis and ovaries are tilted backwards. Intercourse may also be painful when a woman has decreased vaginal lubrication or difficulty becoming aroused due to fertility medications. One over-the-counter vaginal lubricant that is safe to use during infertility is Pre-Seed. You may want to use saliva, egg whites, or mineral oil if you need extra lubrication.

Anna and her husband, David, have been seeing a reproductive endocrinologist for the past two months. She says:

> *I went for an appointment with my infertility doctor yesterday morning. I had blood drawn, a pelvic exam, and a vaginal ultrasound. My doctor suspects I have endometriosis because my menstrual periods are painful with heavy bleeding. I need to schedule laparoscopic surgery for my doctor to view my pelvic organs and laser any endometriosis that is found. I have never had surgery and I worry about what the doctor will find.*
>
> *Last night, my husband wanted to have sex, and I had absolutely no interest. My arm was sore from blood work. I still had gel in my vagina from the pelvic exam and ultrasound. To say the least, I wasn't feeling very sexy.*

At first, he had a hard time understanding why I wasn't in the mood for sex, but after I explained my feelings and my day in the doctor's office, he was very sensitive. He rubbed my back, kissed me, and said how much he appreciated all I go through to try to get pregnant. I am lucky to have such a special husband.

You are the only one who knows your sexual desires. Your partner will need your help understanding how your sexual thoughts, feelings, and responses change during infertility. A man reports feeling less masculine and a woman reports feeling less feminine when achieving pregnancy is difficult. These are only feelings. You are not less masculine and you are not less feminine while you are being treated for the disease of infertility. Communicating your sexual desires to your partner is the key to deeper intimacy in your relationship. Practice talking to each other about your sexual life in an open and accepting manner. These talks are more productive when you are both feeling rested, calm, and balanced. These talks should be delayed if you are feeling sexually frustrated, angry, or upset.

Some couples seek counseling for assistance in discussing how their sex life can be more pleasurable and satisfying. If so, find a counselor who understands infertility and its effects on sexual desire and performance. If you have difficulty talking about sex with your partner face to face, try talking in a dark or dimly lit room, or dialog through writing. Tell each other what you like most and least about your sex life. Be specific and give details. For example, say, "When you kiss me softly on the neck for a few minutes, I get excited and am in the mood for passionate kissing and foreplay."

Men and women usually have different sexual desires at different times during a monthly cycle. These differences can become more apparent during infertility. A woman is more interested in sex when a man makes romantic gestures that help her feel special and loved. A man is more interested in sex when a woman makes sexual overtures and comments about her sexual desire for him.

Adam and Valerie are a couple in their late thirties. This is a second marriage for both of them and they started trying to get pregnant on their honeymoon. After eight months of trying on their own, they were referred to an infertility specialist for treatment. Adam scheduled a couples counseling session to talk about their decreased interest in having sex. He says:

> *Our marriage is how marriage is supposed to be. We got it right the second time around. We are soul mates and best friends. Our sex has always been great until these last two months. Infertility is becoming stressful and taking more of our time, attention, and money. I have to remember that when Valerie is sad and wants to be close to me, she often just wants me to hug her, kiss her, and tell her how much I like her sexy body. This comforts and reassures her and some nights this is all she wants. In fact, it has become what she wants most nights for the past two months of*

infertility treatments.

I want our touching and kissing to lead to intercourse and it's hard for me to slow down once I'm excited. I have no idea how long we will continue trying to get pregnant. I don't want us to settle for an average sex life and I want us to get help with this before it becomes a problem.

Adam's sexual concerns are quite common, and there are many ways to address the problem. It is important to talk about what is happening sexually and how you feel about it. Change begins as you try new ways to respond to each other. Talk about who initiates sex and whether you prefer the initiation to stay the way it is. If not, take turns initiating sex and as you do this, ask your partner what you can do to best arouse him/her.

Remember that sex is mental and emotional, as well as physical. Be aware of the energy level of you and your partner before initiating sex. If you are busy all day and feel depleted at night, you are not likely to have additional energy for sex at bedtime. Maybe waking each other up in the morning after a restful sleep would be a better time for sex. You both need to eat lunch during the day, so meet at home for a "quickie" before lunch. Changing the routine of when you have sex and where you have sex can be arousing.

There are times in every relationship when one partner is interested in sex and the other is not. Sometimes you can stimulate the other person's interest by flirting, giving sincere compliments, and initiating foreplay. At times you may be willing to have sex because pleasing the other person is more important at that moment than your low sexual interest. It is also okay to say "no" to your partner sometimes and expect your partner to accept "no" and be sensitive to your needs. These compromises are important and necessary in all relationships. But any couple, whether undergoing infertility treatment or not, risks decreasing their intimacy and connectedness if they go for weeks without having sex—unless they both agree they want infrequent sex.

Having regular sex is good maintenance for a marriage and keeps your relationship healthy and working well. The longer you go without having sex, the less interested you may become. Remember when you were dating your partner and you felt the excitement of being attracted to each other. Couples who are not having regular sex feel less attracted to each other and they are in danger of settling for a "comfortable" and less passionate relationship. You can settle for having infrequent sex or you can share the joys and pleasures of having a more spontaneous and connected sexual relationship.

You and your partner are the only ones who have the capacity to limit your sexual imagination and creativity. Share with your partner what brings you sexual pleasure so he/she can please you the way you want to be pleased. Note that certain ways your partner touches you at one time may be stimulating, and the same touch at another time can be irritating. This is especially true for women's bodies, so communication is important. You can let your partner know where you want to be touched by moving his/her hand or body part to a particular spot on your body. Try to use words such as, "I would like more of this or less of that," when coaching your partner about what arouses you. You can also demonstrate for your partner how you want to be touched by touching yourself as your partner watches and learns.

There are a multitude of ways you can let your partner know you are interested in him/her throughout the day. This can be done in a sensual or provocative way through phone calls, text messages, or e-mails. Flirt with each other several times a day. Remember to give affection to your partner by how you look at each other and by gestures of touch. For example, when you leave for work, hug your partner, look into his eyes and kiss his lips, rather than inattentively pecking him on the cheek. Bring home a gift, a nice dinner, flowers, or a card for no reason other than to let your partner know you are thinking about her and love her.

These gestures are appreciated when they are least expected, so think romantically beyond Valentine's Day and special occasions. Build anticipation of sex by telling your partner in the morning to be ready for a fun night of sex play, or mention a sexual pleasure he/she should expect to receive later.

You will need to set aside time to relax and have intimate contact. Allow at least one hour to connect, touch, and experience sexual pleasure together. Create a physical environment that stimulates your interest in sex. Have dim lighting or candles in the room. Put blankets and pillows on your floor and lie in front of a fire. Play relaxing music. Turn off all phones and the TV so you will not be distracted or interrupted. Buy massage oil and give each other foot massages, back massages, or full-body massages.

You might increase your interest in sex by going to a book store and buying a book about sex to read together. You may enjoy sharing fantasies or looking at erotic pictures or movies. Wear sexy clothing if that is something you or your partner enjoys. Take as much time as you need to explore each other's bodies and increase your sexual desire. Practice taking turns giving pleasure and receiving pleasure. Lovemaking does not have to include erections, intercourse, or orgasms. It can be done with mouths, fingers, hands, and using any part of your body to relate intimately.

There is an exchange of energy that magically occurs when two people love each other, touch, and intimately share their bodies. This magic goes beyond words and is felt and understood by both partners. At these times, you are reminded of why you chose each other and why you want to build a family together. Sharing the joys and pleasures of sex calms some of the frustrations of infertility. Remember to take time to touch each other often throughout the day. Touching is a simple gesture and takes care of many wants and needs in a relationship. It provides comfort and deepens your connection during this difficult time in your family-building journey.

Chapter 8

Unexpected Gifts for the Spirit

Your infertility experience has the potential to change your life in profound ways. The difficulties of infertility invite you to look within yourself and explore what is meaningful in your life. You may begin a spiritual journey as you connect more deeply with your soul. You will be reevaluating relationships with your partner, your family, and your friends and letting go of old patterns and behaviors that no longer work for you. Some people find that this internal exploration leads you to connect with a Higher Power, God, or a source or spiritual being that is greater than you.

It is helpful when couples and individuals have faith in the Divine, which is anything that brings you closer to understanding that there is a power higher and greater than you. Ask your Higher Power to give you wisdom and guide you through this journey. Trust that your Higher Power is at work in your life and will provide you with courage, strength, and clarity to make choices that are exactly right for you. Spirituality can give meaning and purpose to your struggles, and relying on your Higher Power can help you transcend the hardships of infertility.

If you already have particular religious or spiritual beliefs, they may become more solid. On the other hand, you may be feeling angry towards your Higher Power for allowing this to happen. You may have been praying for a baby and feel that your prayers have not been answered in the way you want. You may not want to attend services in a formal place of worship, a church or a synagogue where families, pregnant women, and babies congregate. Try attending a later worship service where you are less likely to be with babies and families.

If you are having religious or spiritual struggles, use them to help you define what is meaningful and important in your life. Consider meeting with a religious or spiritual mentor who can provide insight, wisdom, and comfort. How you change and how well you manage infertility is entirely up to you, but turning the outcome over to your Higher Power can replace your worry and fear with comfort and peace. These opportunities for growth and change are gifts of infertility.

Kelsey has miscarried three pregnancies during this past year. She says:

> *I am changing as I go through infertility, and this is a lot of hard work. I am appreciating the many blessings I have in my life. I am closer to my husband, more compassionate, and closer to God. I am more aware of my spirituality. I am opening to new things I thought I would never consider before. I am finding a positive connection to every child I see, and I am opening my mind to the possibility that this child may be adopted. It helps me think about*

parenting an adopted child. I knew there would be pearls in this, and now I'm seeing them.

The gifts of infertility unfold as you embrace this opportunity for growth and transformation. Some of these gifts may not become apparent until you reach a resolution to your family building quest. Perhaps the greatest gift of infertility is this unique opportunity for personal metamorphosis and a deeper connection with your Higher Power.

Beliefs

Your beliefs are changing constantly and are influenced by new ideas and experiences. You have probably read a book or had a conversation with someone who influenced you to change a belief. Perhaps as a child you feared you could never learn to ride a bicycle. Then you practiced, learned new skills, and over time you could successfully ride a bike. Your beliefs changed. In a similar way, you are capable of changing the beliefs you have about your infertility. You create negative beliefs when you say, "I will never get pregnant. Why me? Life isn't fair." This negative self-talk leaves you feeling hopeless and defeated, and drains your energy.

You can change your negative beliefs to positive beliefs. One way to do this is by telling yourself, "I am fertile. I will get pregnant. I will carry a pregnancy full term. I will be a parent." For example, Jessica, a client of mine, chose to start thinking of herself as "fertile," rather than "infertile." Several times each day she would sing the words, "I am the Goddess of Fertility." This image of seeing herself as a fertility goddess humored her and helped her feel more empowered in her femininity and fertility.

Are their particular beliefs about your fertility you would like to change? If so, what are these beliefs and what do you want them to become? Write them down and say them out loud several times a day. Post them around your home as helpful reminders that you are incorporating these new beliefs into your reality. In addition, you feel better when you believe that you will get pregnant and have a baby. When deciding on a particular medical treatment, you ask your doctor what the chances are for success. If you have a 30 percent chance of getting pregnant after a particular treatment, why not choose to believe the odds will be in your favor? You have no idea whether you will be in the 30 percent range or the 70 percent range, but you will feel better assuming your treatment will be successful.

Try this exercise when you have fifteen minutes to be still and quiet. Sit upright and close your eyes. Take a few slow and deep breaths and begin to relax. Pay close attention to your body, your feelings, and your thoughts. Imagine your body being as fertile as it can possibly be. For example, create a picture in your mind of you having a large pregnant belly, many active sperm, or several mature eggs ready to ovulate. Let your entire self feel fertile. Stay with this feeling for five minutes. Then stand up, walk around, and move to a chair in another room. Try the same exercise but imagine your body as being infertile. Do you prefer to think of your body as fertile or infertile? What feelings do you associate with each?

Attitudes

Sandra writes about the positive attitudes she and her husband, Christopher, developed during infertility treatments:

> *My ultimate vision for getting pregnant never included stirrups in the doctor's office. I was sad and mad about it for a couple of months. By the time I got my final intrauterine insemination, I was emotionally prepared for it. My husband was in the room with me during the insemination. The doctor came in with the washed sperm. After the insemination, my husband stayed in the room with me and held my hand. We prayed for peace of mind while I remained lying down for twenty minutes. Then we went out to lunch together. It was as fun and romantic as an intrauterine insemination can be. The good news is that we could also go home and have sex afterwards. My husband has a good sense of humor and he is a sensitive and thoughtful person. For two weeks after the IUI, he talked to my stomach and encouraged our embryos to stick around and implant.*

Closely examine the attitude you bring to your infertility experiences. Your attitude comes from within you, and you can choose any attitude you want. It defines how you approach life and how you respond to the world around you. One way to develop a positive attitude is to take time each day to be grateful for all your blessings. List your blessings, say them out loud, and give thanks. Wake up each morning and give thanks for a new day. Focus on three ways you are blessed in your life and give thanks. This sets a positive tone for your day. Go to bed each night giving thanks for three particular blessings you received during the day. This ends your day with positive thoughts and mentally prepares you for a peaceful sleep.

Candace has been noticing her attitude during infertility treatments. She writes:

> *I am working on having a good attitude. Something has shifted for me. I used to think this wasn't going to work, and I would never get pregnant. Now I believe I will get pregnant. There is no reason for this change. I started telling myself I would get pregnant, and now I believe it. I feel more optimistic and hopeful. This is a shift for me, and I know I am different.*
>
> *For our fifth wedding anniversary, we've decided to have fun and blow off treatment for a couple of months. We are taking our first two-week vacation and can't wait. Instead of spending my evenings on infertility Web sites, I'm now going to travel Web sites. I have started think-*

ing of infertility as a marathon and not a sprint. I need to pace myself, take vacation breaks, and trust that I will eventually cross the finish line.

The Present

Infertility can leave you feeling powerless because you cannot control the timing of when life begins or when life ends. You can find comfort and strength believing that a greater plan is at work as you search to become a parent, and that everything happens in life for a reason. When you are in the midst of infertility, the reasons seem unclear and you feel lost in the confusion. You have no idea how your family-building journey will unfold and your future is unknown. A challenge in life, and particularly during infertility, is staying in the present. You only have this moment in time. You cannot change your past, so let it be over and done. You cannot predict the future, so agonizing over something that may never happen isn't necessary.

If you spend your time worrying about what tomorrow may bring, then you will miss today. Slow down and tune in to what is happening around you and within you. Notice the sights, smells, sounds, and textures that surround you. Notice how others love and care for you. Tune into your body and the physical sensations. Notice your feelings and thoughts as they come and go.

Grief

When life is smooth and comfortable, you rarely need to go inward and explore the substance of who you are. The pain and grief you experience during infertility help you become aware of hidden parts of yourself. The grief with infertility is an invisible loss and our culture does not understand or honor invisible losses. In fact, our culture honors a person who is grieving the death of a loved one for only a brief period of time.

In the past, if you were grieving the death of a family member, a woman wore black clothing and a man wore a black arm band. This was a reminder for people to be respectful of your emotional pain, and you were not expected to be cheerful, socialize, or maintain a high level of functioning at home or at work. People would know to treat you with special care during this difficult time. Once your grief subsided and you were ready to resume normal activities, you announced this to others by no longer wearing black.

Today when someone close to you dies, you are allowed to miss work to attend the funeral, but you are expected to return to work within a few days and function as usual. Suppressing grief creates detachment from yourself and others and is a source of emotional stress. If your family members and friends do not understand your pain and grief, ask them to imagine you wearing black. This image can remind them to treat you with special care during your infertility treatment.

Infertility may be your first encounter with loss in your life, and even though you will have other losses each loss is significant and accompanied by grief. Infertility is the loss of your dream to become pregnant or to carry a pregnancy to term. Starting your menstrual period each month is the loss of a desired pregnancy. Having a miscarriage or delivering a stillborn baby is a loss. If you are not able to carry a pregnancy to term, you may decide to use a gestational surrogate or adopt, and you will experience the loss of pregnancy, labor, and delivery. If you are unable to use your own eggs and sperm to conceive, you may use donor eggs, donor sperm, or donor embryos, and you will experience the loss of a genetic connection to your child.

Each person responds differently during times of loss and grief. No one knows exactly how you feel or what you need while you are grieving your losses. Grief is like ocean waves that come and go. Some waves seem powerful, large, and overwhelming. This is similar to how grief feels in the early stages. Over time, your grief becomes less frequent and less intense, much like the waves that are so small you barely notice their coming and going.

Grief is not something you work through or get over. Instead, you learn to manage it and incorporate it as a part of your being. You will always remember this significant time in your life, and it will not become less important if you have children now or in the future. Grief can catch you off guard and reappear when you least expect it. Memories, feelings, and experiences of infertility resurface and fade periodically throughout your life.

Angela and her husband, Blake, had been through many years of infertility treatment and had a six-year-old son as a result of their earlier treatment. She became pregnant again and had amniocentesis at fourteen and a half weeks. The results came back saying she had a normal, healthy baby boy. When she went for her eighteen-week checkup with her obstetrician, there was no fetal heartbeat, and she required surgery to remove the fetus. The following is a letter she wrote to her baby before surgery:

> *My dear baby boy, it is time to say good-bye to you and this breaks my heart. I just looked at my big stomach, which has brought me so much joy for the past four months. I have loved having you with me and have been so thankful you were sent to be a part of our lives. I have felt you were a special gift from God and we have wanted you for so long. Now you have left us and I don't have a clue why. Why now? Why not earlier before we heard you were a healthy boy? What happened to the healthy boy inside of me?*
>
> *I am sorry we weren't meant to be a part of each other's lives. I am sorry I will have an empty tummy in a few days and can no longer be excited about your pending birth. I no longer need your body to be connected to mine. I give my body full permission to release you and ask that*

I stay healthy and fertile. Go back to God—you have and that must be where you belong for now. I so much hoped you would belong in our family, but this was not meant to be.

I will need time to heal from this pain. I know the pain will pass and one day this may make some sense. It sure doesn't now. I don't think I hurt you in any way. Forgive me if I did. I so much hope that one day I will be pregnant again and experience a normal, full-term, and healthy pregnancy with the right baby for this family. I also hope I won't have to work so hard for it. I worked so hard for you and have nothing in return. I will be left empty and in pain.

Maybe one day you will let me know what happened. I will listen. I assume I will learn and grow from this experience but this is not my choice or method of learning. Sometimes I'm tired of the pain and losses, and I want them to stop. I don't want to live with caution and fear of more loss. I am glad our lives connected even though it was brief. I wish you luck on your journey and me on mine. God bless us all. Good-bye with love – Your mom for a short time.

Grieve as long as you need to and grieve any way you choose. You can cry, scream, beat your pillow, and feel sorry for yourself. You can feel angry, betrayed, scared, hopeless, frustrated, and emotionally vulnerable. Move through your grief at your own pace. Allow yourself to feel what you feel and try not to judge your feelings. Over time, you will learn new ways to cope and feel better. You are building a foundation for managing other losses as they occur in your life.

Quiet Time

You will be exploring your inner self during infertility, and personal exploration is best done in solitude. You need time alone to be quiet as you listen to your inner self. When you are gaining new insight and wisdom, it is normal to retreat from social activities and withdraw. Set aside time to reflect upon who you are and who you want to become through this journey.

You may prefer sitting still in a quiet place to connect with yourself. If you are an active person who is unable to sit quietly, there are many ways to connect with yourself on a deeper level. One way is through nature. Spend time outside in nature and notice the colors, smells, and sounds that surround you. Being near water, listening to water, or fishing can provide a time of solitude. Playing in the dirt by gardening or planting flowers may be exactly what you need. If you are a musical person, listen to calm music, dance slowly, or play an instrument. If you want to sing, try using calm, vibrational sound such as chanting a syllable or a meaningful word. If you are artistic, paint, draw, take photographs, make pottery, and find ways to express your creativity. If you enjoy cooking, experiment with new tastes, smells, and foods in the kitchen.

It is important to step out of your busy world, slow down, and connect with yourself. Your deeper joy and happiness are often found in these moments, and you are reminded that infertility does not make you less than whole.

Chapter 9

Practices for Health and Healing

Yoga seems to be everywhere now and many people have become curious about the health benefits of yoga. It may be confusing to know how to find an experienced yoga teacher who is right for you. Be aware that the competency and training of yoga teachers varies from those who took a one-day training and certification class to those who have been devout yoga practitioners and taught for many years. Sri T. Krishnamacharya was one of the world's most renowned teachers of his time. He modernized the ancient tradition of yoga, and several of the world's leading yoga teachers today were his students. His lineage has continued through the teachings of his son, T.K.V. Desikachar, and his grandson, Kausthub Desikachar. They live in India and teach the therapeutic and healing uses of yoga to their students around the world. The teachers trained in Krishnamacharya yoga are among the finest. There are other excellent yoga teachers; attend classes until you find a teacher who is right for you. This is one way for you to take care of improving your health.

Yoga

Practicing yoga is an excellent way to take care of yourself during infertility and throughout your life. It offers a multitude of physical, mental, emotional, and spiritual benefits. A regular yoga practice will improve your health and sense of well-being. It calms the emotional upsets and the physical stresses. It helps create balance in the whole self, which allows for healing to occur. In his book *The Heart of Yoga*, T.K.V. Desikachar writes that yoga has various meanings, and the most common are: "to come together," "to unite," "to link with," "to be one with the Divine," "to direct the mind without distraction or interference." The purpose of yoga is the union of body, mind, and spirit; this is done using asana, pranayama, and meditation. A yoga instructor teaches poses or postures, known as asanas, to increase strength and flexibility. During an asana, you should be steady, alert, balanced, relaxed, and able to stay comfortable in a posture. Steady breathing patterns should be combined with each posture, and a regulated breathing technique, or pranayama, is most effective when practiced after the asana.

When practicing pranayama, you will gradually increase the length of your inhalations, exhalations, and holding the breath between inhalations and exhalations. For example:

- Inhale 3 seconds, exhale 6 seconds. Do this cycle 4 times.
- Inhale 4 seconds, exhale 8 seconds. Do this cycle

4 times.

- Inhale 5 seconds, exhale 10 seconds. Do this cycle 4 times.
- Repeat each cycle and hold your breath for 2 seconds after each inhalation and exhalation. Do this cycle 4 times.

A yoga practice should be carefully adapted to your particular needs, so the ideal practice is done privately with a teacher. If you are in a group yoga class, your teacher will not be able to adjust each posture to adapt to the individual needs of each student. For example, if your ovaries are sore and enlarged while you are on medications, you may feel uncomfortable doing a posture such as a "bridge pose" that tightens the abdominal muscles near the ovaries. If your teacher is aware of your particular needs and limitations, then doing a "pelvic tilt" may be suggested as a more gentle stretch in your abdominal area. However, if it is not possible for you to work with a teacher individually, locate an experienced teacher in your area who is suitable for your needs.

Several books on yoga are listed in the back of this book under Suggested Reading. They have many easy-to-follow yoga lessons, pose adaptations, and special programs if you want to start practicing yoga on your own. Yoga teaches you to be attentive as you link your breath and body while doing the postures. Your inhalation should continue throughout a yoga posture where there is an "opening" movement. Your exhalation should continue throughout a yoga posture where there is a "contracting" movement.

Your yoga practice should concentrate on unifying your body, breath, and mind. Asanas and pranayama are traditionally practiced to prepare you for meditation. If you are interested in developing a regular yoga and meditation practice, designate a special serene place in your home for this practice. You will need a yoga mat or a soft carpet, and this should be a clean and comfortable space where you will not be disturbed by phones or pets.

In this space you may have a table or altar that displays special meaningful objects such as a candle; a picture of a mentor, teacher, or religious leader; or an inspirational book such as the Bible, the Torah, or the Yogasutras. Each time you enter this special place, you do so with an intention and desire to practice yoga and meditation. If you are not interested in yoga or meditation, you may want to go to this special place to pray or to be quiet and reflective.

Breath Work

The easiest and most important way to take care of yourself is through conscious breathing. Your breath is your life force, and your energy comes from your breath. Breathing is your first act when you enter the world and your last act before dying. Although breathing is an automatic process, most people experiencing stress during infertility have restricted and shallow breaths where the chest barely rises during an inhalation, breath doesn't extend into the abdomen, and the exhalation is not complete. This shallow breathing occurs in the upper chest and often causes shoulder and neck tension.

If you want to feel calmer and less stressed during infertility treatment, pay careful attention to how you breathe. Notice if your breath is deep or shallow, fast or slow, if you breathe through your nostrils or mouth, and if you breathe into your chest and abdomen. Your emotions and thoughts are reflected in how you breathe. The quality of your breath and your state of mind directly influence each other. For example, your breath becomes faster and more shallow when you are excited, and it becomes slower and deeper when you are relaxed. As your breath becomes steady and calm, your body releases stress, your mind becomes more clear and quiet, and you feel more emotionally balanced.

Brent is a woman who came for individual counseling after learning that she had a high FSH level and would need to use donor eggs if she wanted to become pregnant. She was shocked to hear this, was having financial difficulties, and wanted help sorting through her feelings and options. She says:

> *In the beginning of our first counseling session you commented that I talked fast and you could not see me inhaling air between my sentences. You said my body looked tense and the tension probably came from my constricted breathing. You asked me to close my eyes, take a few*

breaths, and notice how I was breathing. I thought this was a waste of our time since I had many topics I planned to discuss during our session. For the next ten minutes you taught me how to practice a slower and more relaxing way to breathe. I was not aware of the tension in my body until I changed my breathing. I have followed your suggestions and practice regulating my breath several times a day. This has helped me feel calmer and now I have something I can do to help me feel better. This is so simple and makes such a difference.

Most people live busy lives and are often rushing throughout the day. This fast pace changes how you breathe, and you will notice shallow, quick breathing when you are rushing. This can become a pattern over time, and your body forgets how to breathe in a normal, healthy way. This is an exercise to practice if you want to practice regulating your breathing:

- Begin by exploring the feeling of your breath as it moves in and out of your nostrils. Unless you have nasal congestion, you can control the movement of your breath better through your nostrils than through your mouth, and nostril hairs aid in filtering the air you breathe.
- Try to keep tension out of your throat by keeping your throat as relaxed as possible. Listen to the soft sound of your breath moving through your throat.

- When you inhale, first fill the chest with air, and then fill the abdomen with air. If you want to feel more alert and energized, extend the inhalation and hold it for a few seconds before exhaling.
- When you exhale, first release the air from the abdomen and then empty the air from the lungs. Gently contract your abdomen as you exhale to help push out all the air.
- Continue to explore the feeling of your breath as it moves in and out of your nose, throat, chest, and abdomen. The length of your exhalation should be equal to or longer than your inhalation. If you ever feel discomfort while breathing consciously, this is a signal to stop forcing the breath and breathe easier.

Learning to consciously regulate your breath is your most powerful resource that affects your body, mind, and emotions. These are breath patterns to practice when you want to change your energy or mood:

- To calm anxiety and relax, simply make your inhalations and exhalations longer than normal, and lengthen the natural pause that occurs between the inhalation and exhalation. For example, inhale for four seconds, pause while holding the breath in for two seconds; exhale for four seconds, pause while holding the breath out for two seconds. Gradually lengthen the inhalations and exhalations as is comfortable, and do this in a steady rhythm for many breaths.

- To increase your energy and become more alert, lengthen your inhalation. For example, inhale for six seconds, pause while holding the breath in for two seconds, and exhale for six seconds. Gradually increase the length of your inhalation and keep the pause and exhalation the same. Repeat this cycle many times.

The more you practice regulating your breath, the easier it becomes to keep your attention focused on your breath when your mind begins to wander. You may want to create positive beliefs by saying affirmations aloud or to yourself as you inhale. Examples of affirmations are:

- My sperm will create a pregnancy.
- I will ovulate healthy eggs each month.
- I will carry a pregnancy full term.

These are examples of five different conscious breathing practices:

1. Keep your attention on your breath. Follow the movement and flow of the breath through your body. Notice your inhalation and your exhalation. Continue for many breaths.
2. Follow your breath as it enters and leaves your nostrils.

Continue for many breaths.

3. Focus on a particular place in your body and send your breath to this place. For example, if your shoulders feel tight, focus on sending your breath to your shoulders. Think of breathing in relaxation and breathing out tension from your shoulder area. Continue for many breaths.
4. Imagine your whole body breathing and your breath flowing in and out of every cell, every muscle, and every organ in your body. Continue for many breaths.
5. Count how many seconds it takes to completely inhale. Hold the breath in for a few seconds. Count how many seconds it takes to completely exhale. Hold the breath out for a few seconds. Remember to make your exhalation equal to or longer than your inhalation. Continue for many breaths.

Meditation

There are many forms of meditation. Explore some of them to find one that suits you. You should not begin meditation until the breath and mind are quiet. Meditation is best done in a sitting position. Although it can be done lying down, you want to stay alert and you are trained to fall asleep when lying down.

It is comfortable to sit on a chair or on a pillow on the floor. Sit in an upright position to straighten your spine. Your shoulders should be relaxed.

You may find yourself feeling restless when you first begin to meditate. As with all things you do, the more you practice meditation, the easier it becomes to sit for longer periods of time and "to direct your mind without distraction or interference." Breath work practices and pranayama are forms of meditation. These are examples of three meditations to try:

- Sit upright in a comfortable position on a chair or a pillow. Place your hands on your knees with palms facing upwards. Relax your shoulders and close your eyes. Take a few slow breaths and bring your attention inward. As you inhale, cross your hands over your chest and visualize loving energy entering your heart. Hold this loving energy in your heart for several breaths. Then exhale and lower your hands back to your knees. Repeat this cycle ten times.
- Sit upright in a comfortable position on a chair or pillow. Place your hands on your lower abdomen. Visualize a fertile energy flowing in and out of your reproductive organs with each breath. Hold this fertile energy in your reproductive organs for a few seconds after each inhalation. Gradually lengthen the inhalation, lengthen the hold after the inhalation, and lengthen the exhalation. Continue for five minutes.
- Sit upright in a comfortable position on a chair or a pillow. Place an object before you that is peaceful and

pleasing to you. It may be an object of fertility. Sit quietly and concentrate on the object. Keep your attention on the object for five to ten minutes.

Visualization

Visualization is also a powerful tool that affects the body and mind. You can visualize how you want to respond or visualize an outcome you desire during infertility treatments. Examples of visualizations you can practice several times a day are:

- A sperm fertilizing an egg to create a healthy embryo
- Your body pregnant
- Yourself as a mother or father

Catherine came for counseling to work through her fear of having blood drawn. She reported that the lab technician had difficulty drawing her blood because the blood would begin to flow and then it would stop. The technician would usually have to draw blood from at least three different places on Catherine's arms or hands to get a complete specimen. This was particularly uncomfortable since Catherine and her partner were going through an in vitro fertilization cycle that required having blood drawn many times. She had tried drinking lots of water before having blood drawn but the problem continued. I asked Catherine to do the following exercise in my office and practice it several times a day:

> *Close your eyes, slow your breathing, and say three times out loud: "I am no longer afraid of having blood drawn. I feel calm. My blood flows easily." Then visualize yourself sitting in the lab chair to have your blood drawn. Your breathing is slow and steady. On the first needle stick, your blood flows easily through your vein and into the specimen tube. You feel calm and pleased with your success.*

Catherine had blood drawn daily for seven days and called me one week later saying, "I am practicing what you suggested and it's working. I am having my blood drawn with no problems. The lab technician was shocked and asked me how this change could have happened. I told her about the affirmation and visualization I was practicing, and she plans to encourage other patients to practice this when they have similar difficulties."

Ellie came for individual counseling for several months while she was trying to become pregnant. When asked what wisdom she had learned to share with others, she responded:

> *My suggestion for others during infertility is to always take care of you. What I mean by this is to never feel guilty about how you feel inside, about what you say or how you might act. Let the sadness in so you can eventually squeeze it out. You have to acknowledge your feelings before you*

can let them go. I started feeling better once I started taking care of myself and doing things that made me happy. I learned to avoid certain situations and venture into others. Be good to people who are good to you and spend time with people who make you feel comfortable.

You are the best person to love and care for yourself. Give yourself the love and compassion you deserve. Take time each day to be quiet, still, and turn inward. Use your coping skills that bring you peace and tranquility when you are feeling stressed. Do at least one thing each day that brings you pleasure. Breathe more consciously, locate an experienced yoga teacher, practice meditation, and use visualization.

You may also find pleasure when you dance, exercise, sing, read, get a massage, play with a pet, have lunch with a friend, have great sex, buy flowers, plant a garden, do volunteer work, laugh from deep within, attend a cultural event, play a sport, cook a healthy meal, or take a nap. Explore various ways to calm your body, breath, and mind so you can develop and maintain serenity while trying to become pregnant.

Chapter 10

Music and Imagery to Enhance Fertility

All humans respond to the vibrations of sound in music. When you listen to music, you may recall memories of times you listened to that music in the past, and you may associate feelings, thoughts, people, places, and various other experiences with the music. I recommend listening to music for pleasure and enjoyment every day of your life. Sing or hum with the music, dance and move your body with the rhythms.

Listen to music you like for enjoyment, but during infertility you can also benefit from the therapeutic and healing qualities of music. If you and your partner listen to music together, the music often triggers similar emotions and physical responses for both of you. The music's vibrations and rhythms create an unspoken connection between two people.

When you are in a very different mood from your partner you can change the intimacy level by listening to music together. Close your eyes and hold hands as you listen to a piece of music or dance together. Play a piece of music you both remember hearing at a fun party or event and notice how your connection with your partner feels closer.

I have found classical music to be the most appropriate and

powerful genre to assist you in changing, growing, and healing through infertility. You may wonder why I recommend classical music rather than rock, country, jazz, African drumming, or New Age music, so I will explain.

Classical music most closely matches the complexities of life with its complexities of form, pitch, tone, rhythm, and texture. It embraces the full range of feelings, from agony to ecstasy. The intentional listening to classical music can elicit feelings from deep within you. It can provide a supportive base for you to explore, manage, and change your feelings.

The tensions and resolutions found in much of classical music closely mimic the tensions and resolutions you experience during challenging times in life. A theme may be repeated many times and in various ways during a piece of classical music, and the theme is well organized and integrated by the time the music ends. This is often absent in New Age music.

The resonance of the sound of the instruments in classical music can move through your body, can linger after a note is played, and can stimulate physical responses within you. Your body responds differently when you listen to music played with a solo instrument as opposed to music played with a full orchestra. Since most of classical music is without words, you have the freedom to listen and respond to the music any way you choose.

Classical music is magical in its ability to change your physical, emotional, mental, and spiritual states. On a physical level, listening to calm music can slow your heart rate, lower your blood pressure, and slow your breathing. Calming music can help you manage pain and decrease stress and tension. These are examples of calming classical music pieces:

Satie: *Gymnopedie No. 3*
Debussy: *Reverie*
Respighi: *The Pines of Janiculum*
Fenzi: *Clarinet Concerto, Adagio*
Bizet: *L'Arlesienne Suite No. 1, Adagietto*
Liszt: *Consolation No. 3*

Music with low tones of bass and cello can be felt in your lower abdominal area. During infertility, listen to music with low tones that surround your reproductive organs with vibrational energy. Examples of classical music with cello are:

Haydn: *Cello Concerto in C, Adagio*
Elgar: *Concerto in E Minor for Cello and Orchestra, Op. III, Adagio*
Vivaldi: *Cello Concerto in B Minor*

On an emotional level, classical music can change your mood and help you access your feelings, including those you keep hidden. These are examples of classical music pieces that elicit cheerful and positive feelings:

Copland: *Appalachian Spring*

Elgar: *Enigma Variations, No. 8 and No. 9*
Debussy: *Arabesque No. 1*
Ravel: *Daphnis and Chloe, Suite No. 2*
Brahms: *Symphony No. I, III, Allegretto*

This is an example of a classical music piece that can comfort you:

Haydn: *Cello Concerto in C, Adagio*

On a mental level, listening to classical music can enhance your concentration and focus, and enable you to recall memories of past experiences. It activates the right side of your brain, which stimulates your creative abilities. It can model the tensions you experience during infertility and allow space for finding your resolutions. Examples of classical music pieces with tension and resolution are:

Barber: *Adagio for Strings*
Rachmaninoff: *Symphony No. 2 in E Minor, Op. 27, Adagio*

On a spiritual level, classical music can stir your soul and enable you to access spiritual dimensions of the universe. It has the ability to take you deep within yourself, reaching parts of you that are in need of healing. Examples of spiritual music pieces are:

Gorecki: *Symphony No. 3, Op. 36*
Gorecki: *Totus Tuus, Op. 60*
Part: *Magnificat*
Martin: *Mass*

Experiment with listening to classical music, such as that played on National Public Radio. Decide what you want to achieve through music listening and choose music that is appropriate for what you are trying to accomplish. For example, if you feel anxious sitting in the doctor's waiting room for an appointment, bring an iPod and listen to calm, relaxing music. This is also helpful when you are being inseminated or having an embryo transferred to your uterus during an in vitro fertilization cycle.

If you are having surgery, bring an iPod and listen to music such as Bach: *Concerto for Two Violins, Largo*, which helps your breath and heart rate maintain a steady rhythm. An operating room nurse once questioned why I wanted to wear headphones and listen to music during surgery. She said, "You will be put to sleep and won't even hear the music." I explained that my body responds to the vibrations of music even when my conscious mind is asleep under anesthesia, and this should help my body in healing and recovering from surgery.

There has always been a connection between sound and imagery, and it is widely used in medicine now. During infertility treatment, the woman will probably have at least one vaginal ultrasound to evaluate the uterus, fallopian tubes, and ovaries. During this ultrasound, a probe is inserted into the vagina and pressed against the vaginal wall to direct high frequency sound waves into the body. The sound waves echo back from the body's fluids and tissues, and changes in the sound's pitch and direction are recorded. These waves are measured by a computer and displayed as a picture on the monitor. In a similar way, I also use sound and imagery in my psychotherapy work with infertility clients. In particular, I use the sounds of classical music to evoke imagery from within the client.

Music-evoked imagery is different from "guided imagery" where the guide has a prepared script telling you what to imagine, and background music may be played while the guide is speaking. If you are interested in locating a therapist in your area who is trained in using the music and imagery I am describing, please refer to the Helpful Organizations in the back of the book.

Music-evoked imagery emerges from within you so each person's imagery will be different. In your mind's eye, you may see images or you may experience a memory, a physical sensation, an emotion, a knowing or sensing while listening to the music. Images may evoke your senses of touch, smell, sound, taste, and sight.

The imagery you experience is powerful in that it can linger with you for days, weeks, and years. Therefore, your imagery is easy to remember and use in your everyday life. What you hear when you intentionally listen to classical music is your personal experience, and the images that are evoked from within you are uniquely yours to own and claim. Your internal imagery seems to provide you with exactly what you need at that moment in time. Therefore, you can experience a wholeness in the balancing and integrating of all parts of yourself.

When I am using music and imagery with individuals, couples, or support groups who are experiencing infertility, I begin the session by talking about what the person, couple, or group members would most like to work on changing. Once the goal for change is agreed upon, I use a technique, such as relaxation or regulated breathing, to focus attention inward. I may give a suggestion for imagery such as "let a symbol or image of fertility appear in your mind's eye." I begin playing classical music that I have carefully selected according to the person's or group's goal for change, their mood, and the music's ability to evoke images from within them.

The room should be quiet so the listener can allow images to appear while the music is being played. After the music ends, each person is encouraged to share the images that were experienced. The images usually have special meanings for this person that help meet the goal for change. I encourage the person to remember the images that appeared from within and to think about the images each day so that they can be used as a resource for change.

This is an example of music and imagery I used during an infertility support group for couples:

The couples were talking about the high level of stress

they were experiencing during infertility. The goal of the music and imagery session was to reduce stress. I asked the group to focus on breathing for a few minutes. Then I suggested that they imagine breathing out stress and tension and breathing in calmness and relaxation. I chose the *Canon in D* by Pachelbel for the music listening piece. I started the music and they sat quietly and listened. After the music ended, we spent time discussing each person's imagery. These were the stress-reducing images of the group members:

Tom – *I visualized finishing my dog house.*

Susie – *I had a rush of good marriage memories and was able to relax.*

Rachel – *I saw myself relieving stress in the bath. I visualized a hot bubble bath, wine, a romantic dinner, and dancing. The stress in my back feels better.*

David – *I visualized a creek in Iowa I used to fish in. I felt at peace with everything. It was so relaxing. It was a place I used to go to get away from things.*

Theresa – *I floated with the music. It got rid of the tension in my neck and back.*

Steve – *I took a surrealistic trip and it was going very fast.*

The group members were encouraged to use their images to decrease stress as needed. For example, I suggested that when David feels stress, he visualize fishing in his creek in Iowa and allow his body and mind to feel peaceful and relaxed during this time.

This is another example of music and imagery I used during a women's support group:

The women were feeling discouraged and fed up with infertility treatments. The goal of the music and imagery session was to feel hopeful and positive about becoming pregnant and having a baby. I said, "Notice any thoughts or conversations you are having in your head. Let these thoughts come and go. Don't judge them, just notice them. You will be taking a journey on a body of water. Notice the temperature, depth, and volume of the water. You may choose an object to help you stay afloat. Begin your journey and notice where it takes you." The music I chose for listening was Mozart: *Concerto for Flute, Harp, and Orchestra in C Major, K, 299, Andantino*. After the music ended, the group members shared the following images they experienced:

Sally – *The present body of water was the beach with deep, dark water. The future body of water was clear blue warm water at the ending of the music. The present is not where I want to be now. I'll hold onto the image of the future.*

Mary – *I ended on an island with waterfalls. It was warm. I saw myself happy on this island with the native children. I felt warmth and happiness. I felt physically fit and am motivated to work out again.*

Tamera – *I saw yellow flowers blooming in the middle of the water, and they took over everything. It felt like something was opening up inside of me. It started opening in my low abdomen and moved through the center of my body.*

Patricia – *I was on the ocean. The waves were little. I was suspended in a vitamin E capsule. It was like a womb and I was floating inside it. The liquid, fluid movement in my life would be to drop my worries.*

Catherine – *I was on my favorite lake. My husband was there. The sun was on his face. We were smiling and happy.*

I encouraged the group members to use their imagery

daily to help them feel hopeful and positive. I suggested they draw a picture of their imagery and display it in their home as a visual reminder.

Using music and imagery during an individual psychotherapy session is somewhat different than with a group. With an individual, I spend more time discussing what the client is interested in changing and defining their current struggle. Instead of playing one piece of music, I play a thirty- to forty-five-minute CD that consists of various pieces of classical music. I choose the music to closely match the mood and energy of the individual. As the individual listens to the music, I sit beside them, giving occasional support and encouragement to explore the images that appear.

This is an example of a ninety-minute music and imagery session I had with Joan, who was preparing for an in vitro fertilization cycle. She wanted to keep from getting uptight and tense during her IVF cycle. She also wanted help with how to cope if this IVF cycle was not successful. She said there was a little voice inside her that said, "This won't work. It's hard work." I asked her to focus on her breathing and turn her attention to the little voice inside her that says, "This won't work." The music CD consisted of various Bach pieces. These are the words Joan said while she was imaging with the music:

The voice says, 'You'll never have a baby. You don't deserve it. You haven't worked hard enough. It's something you'll never have, no matter what you do.' Black, dark, ugly, negative, hateful feelings. It comes from the top of my head and takes over. I want the voice to know I believe I can have a baby and I don't have to work so hard. I'm trying to tell that darkness to recede. I'd like to wipe it out with light and hope. Light and hope feel powerful in my heart. I'm feeling victorious. I picture myself on a horse being a victorious warrior in this battle. I want to fight the infertility battle. A sword is slashing fears, doubt, and depression. God is with me and wants me to be victorious. I keep trying to stab out all those things and remember I have God's power. I am asking God to give me his power. He's pouring it into me like a big pitcher, like gold, going through my entire body. I feel strong. God is putting a crown on my head. It has gold and jewels. I am his child and he'll take care of me. I feel regal. I feel confident and reassured. I am walking with my crown and saying, 'I can have a baby.' I'll keep my sword and slash the fear and worries. My sword won. This is joyful. I feel like dancing. I feel movement in my arms. My heart feels light and joyful. I'm feeling victorious. I'm going to have a baby. I picture myself at my house in the nursery rocking with my baby. I feel safe holding my baby. I want the baby to know how desperately I want it to be here. The baby wants me to know it will come and I won't have to wait forever. I'm still picturing the nursery in our house. I'm joyful but have a desperation that it comes soon. The baby says it's coming and I won't have to wait forever. I can keep the picture of the baby in my head and heart and know that it's coming. My hands know the baby is coming. I can feel myself touching and holding the baby. I'm still holding the baby close and singing to it. The baby loves me and is glad that I waited.

After the music ended, we spent ten or fifteen minutes discussing Joan's images, what they might represent for her, and how she could use them to feel calm during and after her IVF cycle. She was feeling strong, hopeful, and serene. The clear and powerful images she experienced while listening to music would not have occurred during a ninety-minute verbal psychotherapy session.

Julia and her husband, John, had been trying to get pregnant for several years. She was only ovulating every few months, and she was not responding well with oral or injectible medications. She was hoping to have intrauterine inseminations, but this was difficult due to her irregular ovulation. Julia came for a ninety-minute individual psychotherapy session using music and imagery. Her initial focus was on recreating the moment of insemination. The music was forty minutes of spiritually evocative classical pieces. These were her comments as she was imaging to the music:

There is a lot of tightness in my uterus. The music helps it let go. It is slow and lazy. What's the rush? There is a sperm on a direct mission to get to the egg. It knows what it's doing. There is still tightness in my uterus. It's more a stimulation and alertness than a tightness. I feel real fertile. There is more stimulation in my pelvis. It can envelop the sperm and bring it to the egg. I tell my body to be gentle with my uterus. Now there are angels singing to my uterus.

The problem is attaching to the lining of the uterus. I need something like vines to help. My uterus says, 'No vines. Use an image of the lining being thick and fertile.' There are angels singing again. The sperm can use my husband's determination, and the egg can be open and vulnerable. The angels can unite them with love. Angel dust can help move them through the tube (fallopian tube) to the uterus. Everything seems to be happening on my left side.

I can see a little girl coming into our lives. I have a sense this is a gift from God. There is a beam. This soul is going to come from far away…near God. I'm holding a child. My ovary is throbbing. There is a message from God saying, 'I'm so glad you appreciate the gift and miracle of children.' We're all children that are his gifts. He lets go of us to let us come here for a short time. He just observes us here. He is directly involved with all of us but he doesn't always act on it because it wouldn't help us. God is handing this spirit down into my body. My ovaries feel more balanced.

Julia had an LH surge that night after her music and imagery session. She called her doctor's office the next morning and went in for an intrauterine insemination. She said, "That was the earliest ovulation of my entire life. It was on day sixteen of my monthly cycle."

Julia's images gave her hope and confidence that she would get pregnant and have a baby. She was surprised to have a spiritual experience with angels and God, and she was amazed by the physical changes in her body's ability to continue ovulating on a regular and predictable monthly cycle. Although her infertility is now in her past, she calls periodically to schedule a "check up" counseling session. She often mentions the powerful images that have remained with her for ten years, and whenever she remembers her images, she feels the same hope and confidence she felt during her significant session with music and imagery.

Note to the Reader

I hope reading this book has given you inspiration, hope, and new ways to experience infertility. I hope it has inspired you to try new ways of experiencing intimacy and sexual pleasure together. This may be one of the most significant challenges you will face during your lifetime. There will be others. You may be surprised to learn that your life unfolds in many ways you never imagined. Your future will become exactly what it is meant to be. Remember you are never alone in your struggles. You have many helpers to guide you if you choose to call upon them, and they exist in both the physical and spiritual world.

In closing, I leave you with a prayer that I recite many times each day. It supports me through difficult moments in my life, and it connects me to my source of inner peace. I think it speaks beautifully to managing the challenges of infertility. Read it aloud and let it resonate deep within you.

The Serenity Prayer

God, grant me the serenity
To accept the things I cannot change,
The courage to change the things I can,
And the wisdom to know the difference.

Glossary of Terms

This glossary includes terms I use in the book, as well as common infertility terms you may see or hear.

Assisted reproductive technology (ART) – All treatments or procedures that involve surgically removing eggs from a woman's ovaries and combining the eggs with sperm to help a woman become pregnant. The main ART is in vitro fertilization (IVF).

Basal body temperature chart (BBT) – A daily record of body temperature taken with a basal thermometer upon waking in the morning before getting out of bed. Used to help determine a woman's ovulation.

Canceled cycle – An ART cycle when ovarian stimulation was carried out but was stopped before eggs were retrieved or before embryos were transferred.

Cervix – Connects the vagina with the uterus. The cervix remains closed during pregnancy and opens, or dilates, during labor.

Cervical mucus – Mucus produced by the cervix that allows sperm to travel to the uterus and fallopian tubes.

Child-free living – A couple chooses a lifestyle without parenting as a resolution to family building.

Conception – The fertilization of a woman's egg by a man's sperm to create an embryo.

Cryobank – A place where frozen sperm or eggs are stored.

Cryopreservation – The process of freezing embryos, sperm, or eggs to be used in the future.

Dilatation and curettage (D & C) – A procedure in which the cervix is dilated and the lining of the uterus is gently removed by scraping or suction.

Donor egg cycle – An embryo is formed from the egg of a female donor and then transferred to a female recipient who is unable to use her own eggs.

Donor embryo – An embryo that is donated by a couple who previously underwent ART treatment and donated their unused frozen embryos.

Donor insemination (DI) – Sperm from a donor is transferred to a woman's cervix or uterus at the time of her ovulation.

Donor sperm – Sperm produced and donated by someone other than a husband or male partner.

Ectopic pregnancy – A pregnancy where the fertilized egg implants in a location outside of the uterus, usually in the fallopian tube, the ovary, or the abdominal cavity. Ectopic pregnancy is a dangerous condition that needs immediate medical treatment.

Egg – A female reproductive cell, also called an oocyte or ovum.

Egg retrieval – A medical procedure to remove the eggs contained in the ovarian follicles.

Embryo – A fertilized egg in the early stages of development.

Embryo transfer – Placement of embryos into a woman's uterus through the cervix after IVF.

Endometriosis – A condition in which cells that normally line the uterine cavity grow outside of the uterus, usually on reproductive organs. It can cause scar tissue, irritation, and inflammation and often leads to painful menstrual periods and infertility.

Erectile dysfunction – A man's inability to achieve or maintain an erection during sexual intercourse.

Erection – The enlarged, rigid state of the penis when a man is aroused.

Estradiol (E2) – The hormone estrogen produced by the ovaries that plays a role in regulating ovulation and preparing the uterine lining for a fertilized egg to implant.

Estrogen – The most important female sex hormone, produced mainly by the ovaries.

Fallopian tubes – Two tubes that transport the eggs from the ovary to the uterus. Fertilization normally occurs within one of the fallopian tubes.

Fertilization – The sperm penetrates the egg to create an embryo.

Fetus – A developing baby in the uterus from the ninth week after conception to birth.

Fibroid – Muscular tumor that grows in the wall of the uterus. A fibroid tumor may or may not interfere with conception or embryo implantation.

Follicle (ovarian) – A sac on the ovary containing an egg.

Follicle stimulating hormone (FSH) – A hormone produced by the pituitary gland that stimulates the growth of ovarian follicles in women and sperm production in men. It is also found in ovulation induction drugs.

Frozen embryo cycle – An ART cycle in which frozen embryos are thawed and transferred to the woman's uterus.

Gamete – The reproductive cell, either a sperm in men or an egg in women.

Gestation – Pregnancy.

Gestational carrier (gestational surrogate) – A woman who carries an embryo that was formed from the egg of another woman. The gestational carrier should have a legal contract that requires returning the infant to its intended parents after delivery.

Human chorionic gonadotropin (hCG) – A hormone secreted by the placenta during pregnancy to preserve the pregnancy. It is the hormone that accounts for pregnancy tests being positive. It can be injected to stimulate the ovaries to release an egg.

Hysterosalpingogram (HSG) – An x-ray study in which dye is injected into the uterus and fallopian tubes to make sure the uterus is shaped correctly and the tubes are not blocked.

Hysteroscopy – A procedure to view the inside of the uterus.

Implantation – The fertilized egg becomes attached to the lining of the uterus.

Infertility – The inability to achieve pregnancy after one year of unprotected intercourse. Infertility is a disease of the reproductive system, and its causes are almost equal between female and male factors.

Intrauterine insemination (IUI) – A medical procedure that involves placing specially-prepared sperm into a woman's uterus. This is done using a plastic tube, or catheter, when a woman is ovulating.

Intracytoplasmic sperm injection (ICSI) – A technique of injecting a single sperm directly into an egg during in vitro fertilization.

In vitro fertilization (IVF) – The process of removing eggs from the ovaries, fertilizing them in a petri dish in the laboratory, and transferring the resulting embryo into the woman's uterus.

Laparoscopy – A diagnostic procedure using a laparoscope to view the uterus, uterine ligaments, fallopian tubes, ovaries, and abdominal organs. Can be used with instruments to diagnosis and treat pelvic disease.

LH surge (luteinizing hormone surge) – The pituitary releases a large amount of luteinizing hormone to cause the mature egg to release from the follicle. It occurs thirty-six hours or less before a woman ovulates.

Luteal phase – The second half of the menstrual cycle that begins with ovulation and has increased levels of progesterone.

Luteal phase defect (LPD) – Failure of the uterine lining to properly develop after ovulation.

Luteinizing hormone (LH) – A hormone that stimulates a woman's ovaries to produce estrogen and to ovulate. In men, it stimulates the production of testosterone, which is needed to produce sperm.

Menopause – The end of menstruation due to aging or failure of the ovaries.

Menstruation – The shedding of the lining of the uterus that normally occurs about once a month in the mature female and continues until menopause.

Miscarriage (spontaneous abortion) – A pregnancy ending in the spontaneous loss of an embryo or fetus.

Multiple gestation reduction – A procedure that involves reducing the number of embryos that have been implanted to improve the chances of having a healthy pregnancy.

Multiple gestation pregnancy – A pregnancy with two or more fetuses.

Myomectomy – The surgical removal of fibroids, or myomas, from the uterus.

Oocyte – A female reproductive cell, also called an egg or ovum.

Oocyte (egg) retrieval – A surgical procedure using a needle to remove the eggs contained within the ovarian follicle.

Ovarian stimulation – The use of oral or injectible drugs to stimulate the ovaries to develop follicles and eggs. Also known as ovulation induction.

Ovaries – The sexual glands of the female that produce the hormones estrogen and progesterone, and where the mature eggs are developed.

Ovulation – The release of a mature egg from the ovary, usually occurring at mid-point in the menstrual cycle.

Pelvic inflammatory disease (PID) – An infection of a woman's reproductive organs that can cause blockages in the fallopian tubes and scarring in the pelvic cavity.

Penis – The male reproductive organ, through which semen is ejaculated.

Polycystic ovarian syndrome (PCOS) – A condition in which the ovaries have multiple cysts, caused by a hormone imbalance that affects ovulation and fertility. It is also characterized by an excess of male hormones.

Polyp – A nodule or small growth commonly found inside the cervix or uterus.

Postcoital test (PCT) – An analysis of a woman's cervical mucus several hours after sexual intercourse to see whether sperm are present and moving normally.

Premature ovarian failure (POF) – A condition in which a woman's ovaries stop producing follicles or eggs before the age of forty.

Progesterone – A female hormone secreted by the ovaries during the second half of the menstrual cycle. Progesterone thickens the lining of the uterus for implantation of the fertilized egg and helps sustain the pregnancy.

Prostate gland – A gland located just below a man's bladder that secretes fluid to help sperm pass through the urethra.

Scrotum – A sac-like pouch at the base of the penis that contains the testes.

Secondary infertility – Infertility in a woman who has been fertile in the past.

Semen analysis – A lab test used to evaluate sperm quality. It measures sperm quantity, volume, concentration, morphology (shape), and motility.

Seminal vesicle – Two small glands located just behind the bladder in the male that produce most of the seminal fluid.

Sexually transmitted diseases (STDs) – Diseases spread by sexual contact, usually an infection. Chlamydia, HPV, and gonorrhea are common STDs.

Singleton – A single live born infant.

Sonohysterography – A saline ultrasound to determine if there are abnormalities inside the uterus or fallopian tubes.

Sperm bank – A place where sperm are stored frozen for future use.

Sperm cells – The male sex cells (spermatozoa), which are produced in the testes.

Stillbirth – The birth of a fetus after twenty or more weeks of gestation that shows no signs of life.

Testes – Two small glands located at the base of a man's penis that produce sperm and testosterone.

Testosterone – A male sex hormone that is produced in the testes and helps produce sperm. It is also produced in small amounts in the female ovary.

Ultrasound (sonogram) – High frequency sound waves used to show images of internal organs, ovaries, uterus, and fallopian tubes on a screen.

Unexplained infertility – An unknown cause of infertility.

Uterus (womb) – The hollow, pear-shaped muscular female organ in the pelvis where an embryo implants and grows during pregnancy.

Vagina – The muscular canal in the female that leads from the outside of the body to the cervix and uterus.

Varicocele – A varicose, or dilated, vein of the testicles, which may cause male infertility.

Vas deferens – Tube that carries sperm from the epididymis to the urethra.

Additional Sources of Information

HELPFUL ORGANIZATIONS

American Association for Marriage and Family Therapy (AAMFT)
www.therapistlocator.net

- Information on locating a marriage and family therapist and important information to read about a variety of problems facing today's families.

American Fertility Association
www.theafa.org

- A nonprofit organization providing resources for infertility prevention, reproductive health, and family building.

American Society for Reproductive Medicine (ASRM)
www.asrm.org

- A nonprofit organization devoted to advancing knowledge and expertise in reproductive medicine, including infertility, menopause, contraception, and sexuality.

Assisted Reproductive Technology Success Rates: National Summary and Fertility Clinic Reports, U.S. Department of Health and Human Services, Washington, D.C., Centers for Disease Control and Prevention
www.cdc.gov/reproductivehealth/ART/index.htm

- The yearly success rates for ART clinics are available online.

Endometriosis Association
www.endometriosisassn.org

- A national nonprofit self-help organization providing education and support, and research for women with endometriosis.

Fertile Hope
www.fertilehope.org

- A national nonprofit organization dedicated to providing reproductive information, support, and hope to cancer patients and survivors whose medical treatments present the risk of infertility.

Fertility Authority
www.FertilityAuthority.com

- The only Web portal dedicated to fertility: provides tools and information that enable women and men to be proactive about their fertility.

Music and Imagery Therapists
www.TheInfertilityCounselor.com/Resources

- To locate music and imagery therapists trained at Southeastern Institute for Music Centered Psychotherapy.

National Certification Commission for Acupuncture and Oriental Medicine
www.nccaom.org

- Provides a directory for finding certified practitioners in Oriental medicine, acupuncture, Chinese herbology, and Asian bodywork therapy.

Organization of Parents Through Surrogacy (OPTS)
www.opts.com

- A national nonprofit educational, networking, and referral organization that supports infertile couples in building families through surrogate parenting and other assisted reproductive technologies.

Polycystic Ovarian Syndrome Association (PCOSA)
www.pcosupport.org

- Provides education, support, and advocacy for women and girls with the condition known as polycystic ovarian syndrome.

RESOLVE, The National Infertility Association
www.RESOLVE.org

- The national nonprofit consumer organization that provides support and information for people experiencing infertility, and increases the awareness of infertility issues through public education and advocacy.

SHARE, National Share Pregnancy and Infant Loss Support, Inc.
www.nationalshareoffice.com

- An international organization to serve those whose lives are touched by the death of a baby through early pregnancy loss, stillbirth, or in the first few months of life.

Society for Sex Therapy and Research (SSTAR)
www.sstarnet.org

- Provides a sex therapist directory.

SUGGESTED BOOKS AND CDs

Borysenko, Joan, *Inner Peace for Busy People,* Carlsbad, CA, Hay House, Inc., 2001.

- Strategies to reduce stress, create a peaceful mind, and transform your life.

The Dalai Lama and Culter, Howard, *The Art of Happiness*, New York, Riverhead Books, 1998.

- How to find happiness and inner peace.

T.K.V. Desikachar and Cravens, R.H., *Yoga and the Living Tradition of Krishnamacharya*, Aperture Foundation, Inc., 1998.

- An introduction to the life, work, and teachings of Krishnamacharya and his living influence.

T.K.V. Desikachar, *The Heart of Yoga: Developing a Personal Practice,* Rochester, VT, Inner Traditions International, 1995.

- An invaluable source of information regarding the theory and practice of Krishnamacharya yoga.

Hay, Louise, *The Power Is Within You*, Carlsbad, CA, Hay House, Inc., 1991.

- Ways to learn about yourself, love yourself, and improve the quality of your life.

McCarthy, Barry and McCarthy, Emily, *Rekindling Desire*, New York, Brunner-Routledge, 2003.

- A step-by-step program to help low-sex and no-sex marriages.

Metz, Michael and McCarthy, Barry, *Coping with Erectile Dysfunction*, Oakland, CA, New Harbinger Publications, 2004.

- How to regain confidence and enjoy great sex.

Moore, Thomas, *Dark Nights of the Soul*, New York, Gotham Books, 2004.

- A guide to finding your way through life's ordeals.

Myss, Caroline, *Anatomy of the Spirit*, New York, Harmony Books, 1996.

- The seven stages of power and healing.

Pierce, Margaret and Pierce, Martin, *Yoga for Your Life*, Portland, OR, Rudra Press, 1996.

- A yoga practice manual of breath and movement for both the beginner and experienced Krishnamacharya yoga student. Contains progressive, easy-to-follow lessons, pose adaptations, and special programs.

Skaggs, Ruth, *Music: Keynote of the Human Spirit*, Baltimore, MD, Publish America, 2004.

- An exploration of the profound influence of music on our lives since early human history.

Skaggs, Ruth, *Healing Music*

- A CD that consists of music selections to meet a variety of emotional and physical needs.

To order: www.musicartstherapy.com; go to Finishing Strong Book Ordering Information.

Talmadge, Lynda and Talmadge, William, *Love Making: The Intimate Journey in Marriage*, Saint Paul, MN, Syren Book Company LLC, 2004.

- To help couples enhance their emotional and sexual intimacy.

Tolle, Eckhart, *The Power of Now,* Novato, CA, New World Library, and Vancouver, B.C., Canada, Namaste Publishing, 1997.

- A guide to spiritual enlightenment.

PERIODICALS

Yoga Journal

- Excellent yoga magazine published monthly.

References

Introduction – National Survey of Family Growth, 2002. Centers for Disease Control and Prevention, U.S. Department of Health and Human Services.

Chapter 6 – American Society for Reproductive Medicine (ASRM), 2004. *Fertility and Sterility Journal,* 81: 527-531.

Chapter 9 – T.K.V. Desikachar, 1995. *The Heart of Yoga: Developing a Personal Practice.* Rochester, VT: Inner Traditions International.

Chapter 10 – Ruth Skaggs, 1997. *Finishing Strong.* St. Louis, MO: MMB Music, Inc.

Ruth Skaggs, 2004. *Music: Keynote of the Human Spirit.* Baltimore, MD: Publish America.